S0-AJA-977

The Self-Health Guide

First Printing, 1980

Second Printing, 1981

Third Printing, 1984

All Rights Reserved

Copyright 1980 by Kripalu Yoga Fellowship

Printed in the United States of America
by Kripalu Publications
Box 793
Lenox, MA 01240

Library of Congress Catalog Card No: 80-82166
ISBN: 0-940258-00-5

THE SELF–HEALTH GUIDE

A personal program for holistic living

Compiled by the staff of Kripalu Center for Holistic Health,
based on the teachings of Yogi Amrit Desai.

Contributing Illustrators, Designers and Editors:

Carolyn Delluomo
Lesley Dove
Carol Finnegan
David Jackson
Laura Moore
William Nuessle, Ph.D.
Don Stapleton, Ph.D.
Jane Yelland

Photographs:

All photographs were taken by staff photographers of the Kripalu Center for Holistic Health except the following, which we acknowledge with thanks:

Cathy Leaycraft, pp. 6, 46 (upper right), 179.
Peter Mellon , pp.   3, 123 (lower right(, 138, 146, 161, 186, 191 (lower), 196.

Special Note:

Most photographs are of the grounds of the Kripalu Center for Holistic Health or of program participants at the Center.

WHAT PEOPLE HAVE SAID ABOUT THE KRIPALU APPROACH

"Spending a week at the Kripalu Center for Holistic Health has been a turning point in my life. The experience has had a profound effect on my thinking and, therefore, on how healthy I feel. I realized that I hadn't really taken the time to listen to my body for many years, and when I did I had more control over my health. I learned that when I feel better physically, I feel better emotionally."

Ruth Russ, Grand Rapids, MI
College Music Teacher

"I'm still savoring the experience you and your community provided for me. I'm amazed at how clearly your love shines in so many ways, and I'm inspired to create a living situation for myself which more closely approximates it."

John Travis, MD
Founder, The Wellness Center

"My feelings of well-being and peace with myself have never been so complete."

Frances Harris, Springfield, PA
Business Administrator, University Medical Dept.

"I came with the pleasant expectation of doing some cleansing through fasting and yoga, and achieving greater body-mind-spirit centering. I have achieved that and much, much more, in ways I did not anticipate. I gained a profound inspiration from the Kripalu Approach to living...an enlightenment of my understanding of Holistic Health. What I have been practicing and studying for the past 1 ½ years...has been expanded into an even wholer approach than I knew existed...living the Kripalu way."

Beverly Klayman, Washington D.C.
Secretary

"I learned there is a simple way for me to assume responsibility for my own health and well-being."

Cynthia Stephens, Detroit, MI
Teacher of Emotionally Impaired

"When I came I felt very low in energy both physically and mentally...now I feel so hopeful, optimistic and vibrant, and I'm more in touch with the cognitions and behaviors that led me to lose energy."

Jacqueline Richied, Arcanum, OH
Mental Health Counselor

"I feel tremendous -- the total overall approach to full development and joy is outstanding."

Kathleen Sanwald, Middletown, NY
Teacher

"It is in being able to take home the lessons that my wife and I learned, and use them constructively every day, that places the truest value on the experience of the Health Center. We have learned to eat better, to relax more easily, to face ourselves more successfully within the limits that we have and to enjoy what we attain there."

Roy Harris, Springfield, PA
Aeronautical Engineer

"I've experienced a miracle of healing and self-acceptance, and I'm in a new and wonderful place filled with love and joy. I'm so excited about life; I feel that a new door has opened for me and I'm really just beginning to live."

Bette Naravati, Richmond, VA

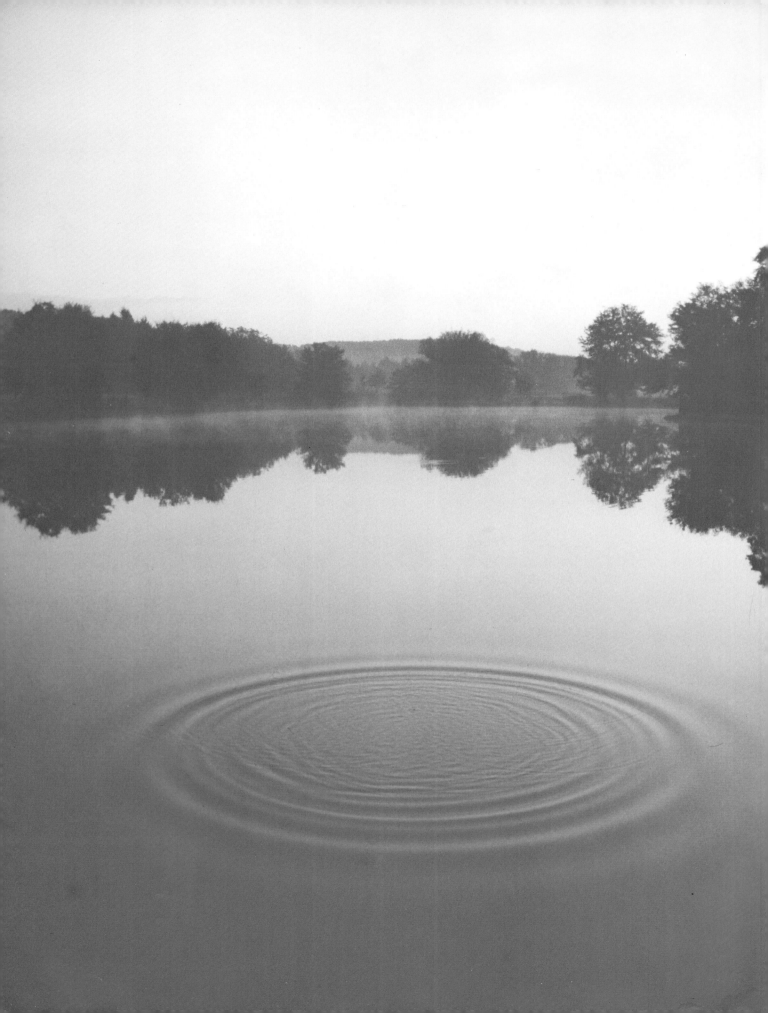

*Your own body is the very best book on health
that you will ever read.*

Table of

Contents

INTRODUCTION
about this book

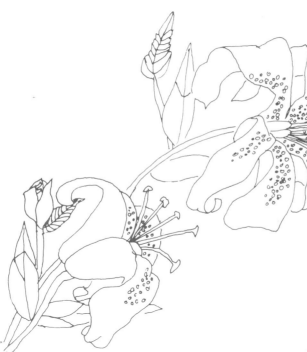

Most books can, at best, significantly add to your store of intellectual or theoretical knowledge *about* life, or *about* yourself. A few unique books are able to give you, in addition, penetrating insights and authentic *experiences* of yourself that go so deep they make permanent changes in the way you experience your life. We believe this is such a book.

THE STRUCTURE OF THE BOOK

This book has been structured in such a way as to make your experience a source of learning. The first section, entitled "The Questions", is based on the premise that to find the right answers from life we must first ask ourselves the right questions. When the right question has been arrived at, by a process of refinement, the seeds of the answer will be found within the question itself.

The second section, entitled "The Answers", outlines the eight ways in which the Kripalu Approach can answer these questions about life and health. Each of these eight "pathways" consists of three basic kinds of material designed to make learning enjoyable, easy, and experiential, rather than purely didactic. These three kinds of material are:

(a) Articles which describe the basic principles and theory of the Kripalu Approach
(b) Self-Discovery Experiences which put you in touch with where you are now in relation to these health principles
(c) "How To" sections which give practical ideas, exercises and techniques to implement what you have learned.

The articles come from two sources: some are adaptations or condensations of talks and lectures given by Health Center Founder-Director, Yogi Amrit Desai; the remainder are compilations of material taught at the Center by the professional staff. The latter are based on Yogi Desai's teachings, but also integrate other sources drawn upon for workshops, sources both ancient and modern, Eastern and Western.

HOW THIS BOOK WAS BORN

This book came into being as a response to a need. Guests at the Kripalu Center for Holistic Health frequently asked us for "something I can take home to continue the work I started here." Then they began to ask us for a book that would enable them to share their experience here -- which they told us was unique -- with friends and relatives who could not come to participate in our programs. And so this book was compiled, at first in workbook form, from our program materials.

The response was so enthusiastic that we quickly sold out, and when the time came for reprinting we decided to expand the material and make it available to a wider public by editing it into a more conventional format. This was a real challenge; how were we to transpose the in-depth, holistic experience of a stay at the Health Center into the traditional, linear book format? Not only that -- how could we freeze in time the material from our programs, which are constantly evolving in an organic way as we learn from both our own experience and that of our guests?

Well, we overcame those obstacles, and the result is The Self-Health Guide. We're excited about it -- and we think you will be too. Because here is a book that has all the ingredients to change your life, just as the lives of visitors to the Kripalu Center for Holistic Health have been changed.

Kripalu "Self-Discovery Experiences"

As we said earlier, reading a book does not, as a rule, put us in touch with our own experience -- more often than not it takes us out of our experience and into intellectualization about it. While intellectual learning clearly has its place in life, in the area of personal growth and development experience is undoubtedly the best teacher. According to developmental psychologists, we learn more in the first few years of our lives than in all of the remaining years, because, at that age, we learn experientially rather than intellectually. This is the first reason for the inclusion of self-discovery experiences.

The second reason is that the Kripalu Approach is based on experiential learning. As a visitor to the Kripalu Center for Holistic Health, you would find that experience is the primary ingredient in the programs. This book has been designed, as we said earlier, to bring you an approximation of the experience you would have if you came here.

The third reason is that personal experiences are just more fun! It is much more interesting and real to experience something for yourself than to simply have it explained to you.

Why do we call them "Self-Discovery Experiences"? Because, very often, most of us simply do not know where we stand in certain areas or what we are really experiencing, deep down where it counts. We are accustomed to not acknowledging our feelings for social reasons

and need practice in getting back in touch. Often we don't even know what we are feeling!

We think that what we think is what we feel. That is why we call these introspections "Self-Discovery Experiences". They are experiences that help you to re-discover yourself: what you really think and feel about life, about health, about yourself. Then you can go on from there to make any changes you may *feel* you need.

One important thing to know about these "experience" introspections: sitting quietly with your eyes closed and really becoming relaxed is very important. Take the time that is needed to do this before you start. It allows the answer to come to you from a subconscious level -- a level beyond your conscious, habitual thinking. As you become more adept at the technique, you will be amazed at what you are able to learn -- from yourself!

This book is intended as a workbook and a fun book for you to record your experiences and discoveries. You may prefer not to write in the book itself, and in places you'll probably need more space (especially where we invite you to draw). So, we recommend that you work in a special notebook or journal, so that the material remains in sequence and does not get separated or scattered as it may if it is on loose sheets. You will find it helpful to be able to refer back to your notes easily as you monitor your progress. Have fun!

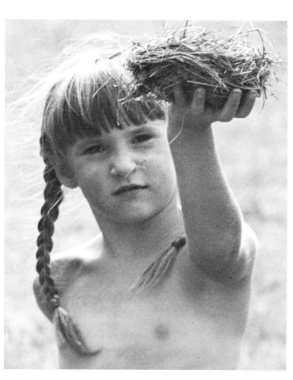

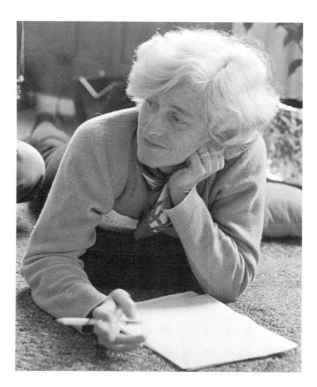

THE THREE "A"S

A key part of our approach to self-discovery is "The Three 'A's": Awareness, Acceptance and Adjustment. These are the three stages into which the Kripalu Approach divides the process of making desired changes in our lives.

1. Awareness. This stage indicates that we must know where we are now before we can decide how to get where we want to go. It's like setting off to drive to see friends, getting lost and having to phone them for directions. Before they can tell you how to get to their house, the first question they must ask is: "Where are you now?" So, for this first stage of Awareness, we must go through the process of seeing clearly where we are now.

2. Acceptance. This is where acceptance becomes necessary. Awareness and acceptance are intertwined. By learning to freely and uncritically accept where we are, whether or not it is where we want to be, we will begin to allow our unconscious to release more and more knowledge about ourselves. So, the process of acceptance is one of simply acknowledging to ourselves that where we are is okay, is fine, is in fact perfect -- it is where we are supposed to be right now. After all, that's the movie that's playing right now, so let's enjoy it! Mentally fighting what is ("I should be better") simply makes us lose energy and self-esteem. Without acceptance of where we are, there is no possi-

bility of going further or of enjoying ourselves fully. Until someone acknowledges that he or she *is* overweight, for example, they will not be able to find ways to lose that weight.

3. Adjustment. Once the two preceding stages have been fully experienced and embraced, we can tranquilly go on to make the changes in our habits that we desire and that will bring us to a state of greater holistic health.

The keys to the stage of Adjustment are patience and moderation. Often, we either want to go too far too fast and become discouraged when we can't change everything overnight, or else we feel that the changes needed are so great we'll never be able to do it, so we are discouraged from even starting. The Kripalu Approach recommends gentle, gradual, easy-to-accomplish changes, starting with something we know we will find pleasant and not difficult. Then, encouraged by our early success, we'll feel inspired to continue into slightly more difficult areas without becoming discouraged. In other words, the whole process is a game we play with the subconscious mind, tricking it into giving up its grip on our old, non-productive habits. These three steps of Awareness, Acceptance, and Adjustment are used in each of the eight paths to health in the Kripalu Approach. In fact, they can be used to facilitate any of life's transitions, from changing one's job to dealing with accidents or even severe illness. Try them and see.

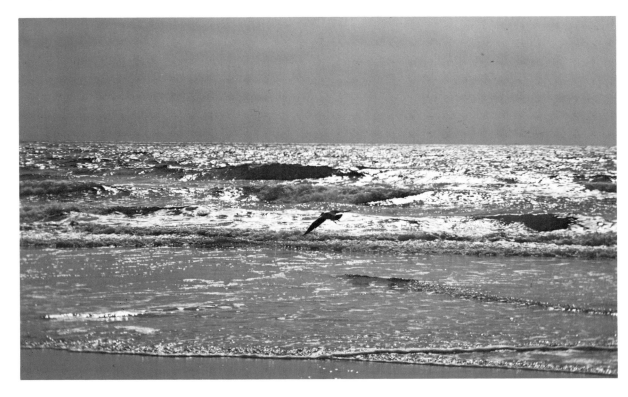

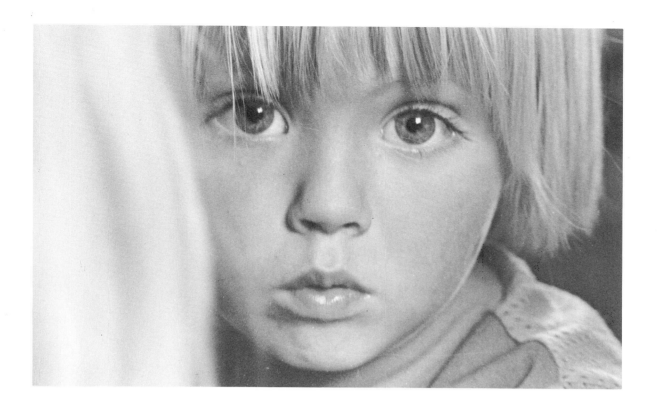

HOW TO GET THE MOST OUT OF THIS BOOK

1. Use it to experience yourself in new ways, not just to add to your store of intellectual knowledge. Buying a cookbook is a good analogy -- you wouldn't just read the recipes, you'd cook them and enjoy the meal. What you will enjoy from immersing yourself totally in this book is a new and exciting experience of yourself that will make your whole life healthier and happier.

2. Digest it slowly, chapter by chapter. Continuing the recipe analogy, read as if you are savoring a delicious meal and want to get the most out of every succulent mouthful. Complete each Self-Discovery portion before going on to the next section of straight reading.

3. Follow the recipe closely. First find a quiet, peaceful, pleasant place to read the book and, especially, to do the exercises, so that you can really take in the material and allow it to affect you on a deep level.

4. Observe the way you are using this book as another part of the learning it can convey to you. Notice whether you have a tendency to want to just continue reading (passive, uses less energy, requires no self-revelation) or whether you are eager to complete the Self-Discovery Experiences (active, requires more energy, reveals you to yourself).

5. Take one step at a time. Select one area at a time where you know you will enjoy working and changing. Make a commitment to changing that one area of yourself and other changes will automatically occur. When you pull a table by one leg, the other three legs come too!

6. Enjoy yourself! More than anything else we want this book to be enjoyable, fun, and a pleasure to read and work with. Getting to know yourself better is the most wonderful experience there is.

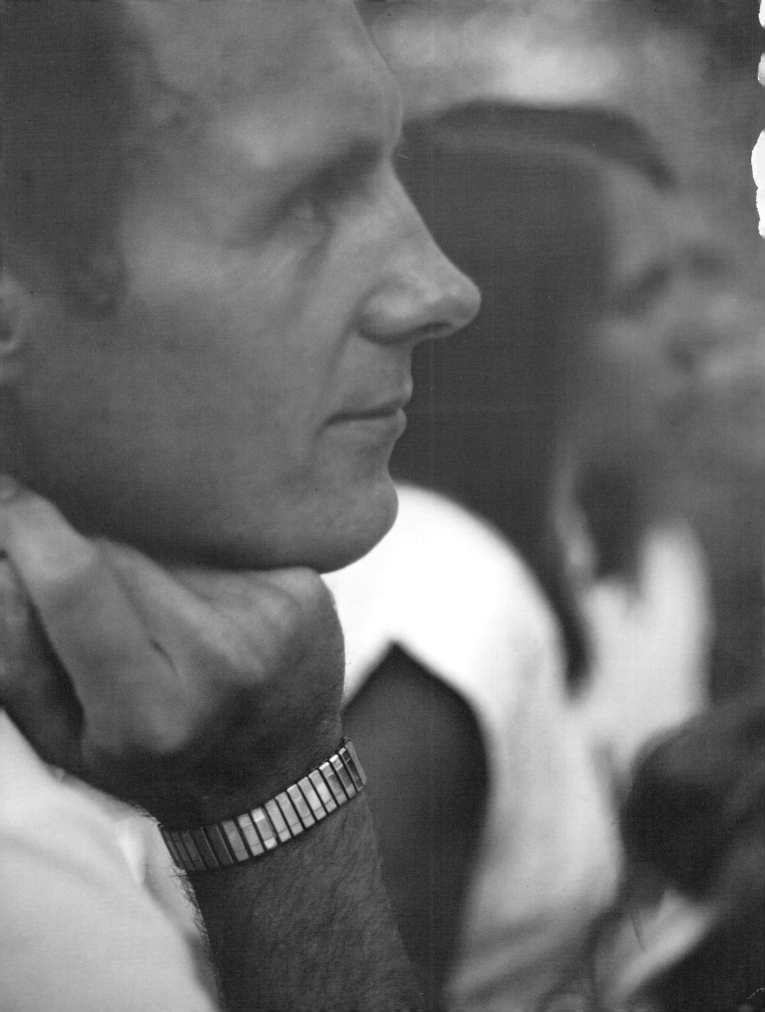

SECTION ONE
the questions

WHAT IS HOLISTIC HEALTH?

Did you know that in the next sixty seconds your heart, which is only about the size of your fist, will pump no less than five quarts of blood around your body, through 60,000 miles of veins, arteries and capillaries? Or that in the space of that same minute, one hundred and twenty *million* new cells will be created for the effective maintenance of your body, without your having to give it a moment's thought? Or do you give it thought?

Since you are reading this book, you are probably one of a growing number of people who are beginning to realize that a greater awareness of the miraculous functioning of the human body can greatly improve the quality of your life and health. Whether you actually know the meaning of the words "Holistic Health" or not, you have already embraced its approach to life: an approach that affirms that there is more to health than mere absence or avoidance of disease, that true health is a state of radiant well-being. Life, to the Holistic Health practitioner, is more than just living; it is a celebration of being alive. It is being captivated by the supreme craftsmanship of nature in the body, mind and spirit. It is coming to realize that the human body, like the violin of a virtuoso musician, is a delicate and subtle instrument which must be handled with the greatest of care and respect and tuned with deep sensitivity before the music of life can pour from it with beauty and harmony.

Holistic Health is a new, yet very old approach to life, which invites us to activate our latent ability to become the artist and creator of our own life and health. It invites us to recognize that, by first creating harmony within our own body, mind and spirit, we can become co-creators in the great symphony of life, and not merely hum a pleasant but mediocre melody. Holistic Health invites us to affirm nature's miraculous artistry in us by attaining the high level of radiant health, inner peace and joyful spiritual well-being for which we were born.

Whole, Hale and Healthy

Most of us have grown up with a limited perception and definition of health. Even our modern dictionaries define health as: "the condition of being sound in body, mind or soul; especially freedom from physical disease or pain " (Webster). If you take a minute to look more closely at the roots of the word, however, you see something more. "Health" comes from the Old English word "Hal", which means whole. "Holy", the condition "characterized by perfection and transcendence" (Webster) also comes from this root. They, together with the word "holistic" or "holism", have a common ancestry in the primal Greek root "holos", which means whole. The basic perception suggested is that health means being whole. It involves all that we are. We therefore shortchange ourselves if health is perceived merely as the physical state of not feeling ill. The currently emerging approach of Holistic Health is an effort to experience what the Greeks had in mind long ago: the experience of wholeness, a wholeness that borders on "hol-i-ness"; body, mind and spirit in a triune affirmation of our fullest health potential.

Yogi Amrit Desai, in a recent lecture to helping professionals, summed up the holistic approach as follows: "awakening the body to its higher potentials, in cooperation with a healthy mind, is the beginning of Holistic Health. In this awakening there naturally emerges an awakening of the higher consciousness within you."

Such a definition of health is much beyond the scope of a successful physical exam and could hardly be measured by it! The question is, are we willing to broaden our image of health and affirm that, "Yes, health is more than the absence of disease; it is more than eating right, quitting smoking, or jogging everyday. It involves all I think, feel, say and do. It is the harmonious interaction of all parts of me: my body, mind and spirit. It is holistic. My well-being rests in my ability to affirm that all of me is involved in the experience of feeling good. And in that involvement of the totality of who I am, health becomes not just maintenance, but a celebration of my self, my universe, my life."

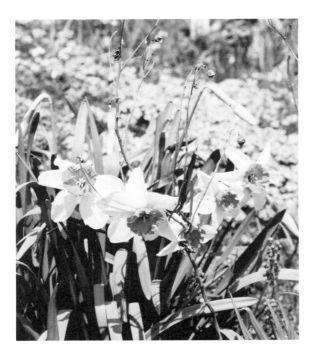

Settling for Second Best

When you begin to examine your definition of health and the degree to which your actions are consistent with your definition, you may find that unconsciously you have been settling for second best. You may discover that though you believe true health to be the experience of vibrant well-being, you've been settling for a level of well-being that simply involves the absence of disease.

Many of us grew up believing that we "catch" a cold and we should "cure" our ailments by taking medication. We unconsciously subscribe to a definition of health that merely maintains life, rather than celebrating it. These actions and perceptions have their roots in the traditional model of health care in which most of us have been raised. Since the time of Louis Pasteur, in the mid-1800's, the model for health care has been the microbiological interpretation of disease. The "germ theory", which demonstrated the existence of germs and their relation to disease, began to find its way into our medical systems and mode of life. The interpretation of health became dominated by the belief that if germs could be controlled, suppressed or destroyed, then the consequent experience was one of health. The result is a second-best definition of health. "I am well if I'm not ill and if my doctor says so."

Hygea and Panacea

Even in ancient Greece there were two schools of thought that philosophically reflected both the traditional and the holistic models of health. The goddess Panacea ruled over the domain of healing and represented the approach of making a wrong (an illness) right, while Hygea was the goddess of health through appropriate living. The holistic approach suggests a return to the domain of Hygea, of enjoying health by involving all our energy -- physical, mental and spiritual -- in living in harmony with the laws of nature.

Take a look now at the chart (Fig. 1) which compares the holistic and traditional models. Notice the actions and perceptions that most closely approximate your own steps toward health. Notice the claim of holism that it is not merely a germ that is responsible for our lack of health and it is not our physician who is responsible for making us healthy. It is we, ourselves, who are ultimately responsible for the level at which we are in harmony with the health-sustaining laws of nature. Though another may offer guidance, tips, formulas, cures, it is *I* in the last analysis who am the vehicle through which this energy of life flows. It is *I* who create the inner and outer environment in which the light and health can shine.

Fig. 1
A Comparison of the Traditional and Holistic Health Care Models

TRADITIONAL HEALTH CARE	HOLISTIC HEALTH CARE
Looks at diseases and symptoms	Looks at whole person
Cares for body and mind	Cares for body, mind and spirit
Aims at normal health, i.e. absence of disease	Aims at high-level vibrant energy
Symptoms of body and mind treated by separate specialists	Integrates treatment of body, mind and spirit
Focuses on treatment & cure	Focuses on prevention & education
Is for crisis intervention	Is for ongoing maintenance of health
Based mainly on drug or surgical intervention	Based on natural methods of restoring balance wherever possible
Based on theory and scientific proof	Also accepts experiential and intuitive approaches
Sees patient as passive, unknowledgeable recipient of cure	Recognizes individual's right and ability to take responsibility for own healing process
Based on traditional Western allopathic methods	Also utilizes non-traditional, non-Western and homeopathic methods

9

WHAT IS THE KRIPALU APPROACH?

The Kripalu Approach is based on two fundamental principles. The first is that expressed in the opening quote of this book: "Your own body is the very best book on health you will ever read." These words were spoken by the founder of Kripalu Center for Holistic Health, Yogi Amrit Desai. He went on to ask: "But do you know how to read it?" The Kripalu Approach teaches us how to read it; how to focus our attention on our own experience of our bodies, and then learn to interpret that experience and use it as our own personalized path to vibrant health and well-being. We thus begin by turning inward, observing ourselves and seeing the ways in which we have experienced our lives so far.

Next we are asked to make a strong affirmation, to say, "I accept my present state of health and well-being, with its weak spots. I recognize that I have created my health, consciously or unconsciously, and I take responsibility for it. I create my life's experiences, and where I am right now is exactly where I need to be to learn about life and health." We cannot take steps in any new direction until we know the ground on which we are standing, until we harvest the wisdom that comes from the lessons of our own experience thus far.

The second basic principle of the Kripalu Approach is that we need to see our lives and health in a new way, as expressions of energy. Everything that we say and do is an expression of our own inner life energy, of spending it or conserving it.

Our present state of well-being is a result of how wisely we have used that energy in the past. There is no question of being self-critical here, or of judging the way we used our energy as good or bad. We simply did what we could with the awareness that was available to us at the time. Now, however, we can learn to see our lives in a new light, in terms of energy. To do this, we need to understand what the Kripalu Approach calls the "prana principle".

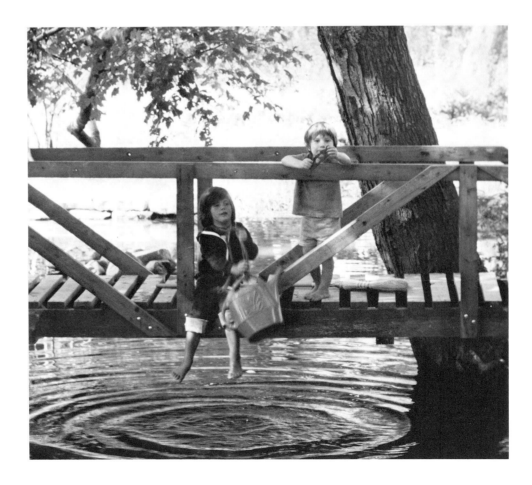

WHAT IS THE PRANA PRINCIPLE?

The wisdom on which our life depends has never come to us as verbal information. This wisdom is the wisdom of PRANA, the life force within us which activates all the functions of the body. Guided by its own innate intelligence, prana flows through the nerve currents of the body as a conscious energy and carries out millions of intricate life-giving processes with precise order and intelligence. This wisdom is known by many names: body instinct, wisdom of the body, inner voice, involuntary nervous system, intuition and inner guidance. Whatever name we choose, the wisdom of prana is far superior to any other knowledge that we have today. Even in this age of advanced science and technology, we have failed to fully comprehend or reproduce that which prana accomplishes daily within our bodies. We never had to learn how to breathe, circulate our blood, digest our food, eliminate our poisons or heal our bodies, because the life force of prana, with its unparalleled and often incomprehensible innate intelligence carries out all such complex processes for us from birth to death. Ignoring this inner wisdom is the root cause of all disease; listening to its unerring advice is the best program of Holistic Health available to us.

This is how Yogi Amrit Desai describes prana. Prana is the inner energy, the individual manifestation of the life force, that accomplishes our essential life functions without our having to do anything consciously. But prana can also help us to accomplish correctly the life functions which are not automatic, which require us to make conscious decisions: when and how much to eat, to sleep, etc. Prana "speaks" to us through our intuition, our inner sense of knowing what is right or wrong for our body at any given time. Yet we have learned to ignore it, and sometimes do not even feel it. It has become a lost language which we have completely forgotten how to read. We have all experienced those moments when we sat down to a meal and ate because it was delicious, not because we were hungry. By so doing, we ignored prana. Or perhaps one night we were very sleepy, but a friend called and we went to a movie anyway. Our tiredness was prana's way of speaking to us, saying we needed sleep. Again, we ignored prana.

If we do not listen to prana, we miss the opportunity of experiencing the balance and inner harmony that is our birthright. At minimum, we do a disservice to our body as well as to our whole being. If done habitually and often enough, we create the state of dis-ease in the body, a disharmony between and within body, mind, emotions and prana. When our prana is depleted, we become restless and negative in our outlook on life. Our imagination becomes limited; our creativity is impaired; we cannot think clearly. We have no zest, no energy, no vitality. Faced with this condition, prana will seek to fulfill its natural role of homeostasis, of restoring us to "ease", but it is only our listening and response which will make the healing possible.

Thus the source of our health is nowhere else but within us. We can read all the books on health, but they won't help much until we know how to read our own bodies and the signals of prana. In this way, illness becomes our messenger, a telegram telling us that somewhere in our lives we have lost balance. Prana can be a diagnostic center within us, our own Holistic Health handbook. The purpose of the Kripalu Approach is to learn how to attune to prana, to listen to the wisdom of the healer within us.

Holistic Health teaches that health does not end with having a finely tuned body, nor does it end with also having a calm, perceptive mind. It culminates in the experience of the merger of all aspects of ourselves: body, mind and spirit.

HOW CAN I USE THE PRANA PRINCIPLE?

When the inner life energy, the prana, begins to become active through the practice of holistic techniques, a unique phenomenon occurs. Our own vital energy, the innate intelligent force within us, begins to correct physiological and psychological blocks lodged within the system. We begin to establish a direct form of communication with the healing force within us. We tap our true nature.

Yogi Amrit Desai

This communication is the re-establishment of contact with our intuition, our inner knowledge of what is right for us as whole, integrated beings. By progressively allowing the evolutionary force of prana to guide us, we have the potential to reach to the apex of our energy, a transcendence of normal well-being.

The chart entitled, "Levels of Health" (Figure 2) symbolizes our growth, through prana, toward true well-being. Health is not truly holistic unless and until it encompasses an ascent towards this realm of self-realization. Figure 2 portrays the significance of this perception and definition of health. At its lowest level, health is simply a matter of avoiding death and moving towards a "normal" combination of sickness and health. Also the focus is mainly on the physical body.

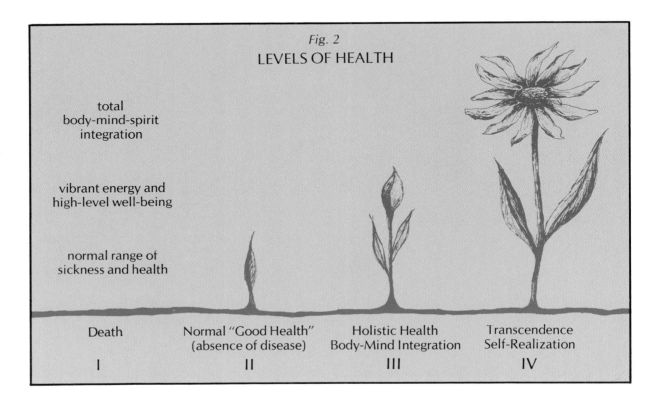

Fig. 2
LEVELS OF HEALTH

total
body-mind-spirit
integration

vibrant energy and
high-level well-being

normal range of
sickness and health

Death	Normal "Good Health" (absence of disease)	Holistic Health Body-Mind Integration	Transcendence Self-Realization
I	II	III	IV

Rising above this level of defining health, we come to a positive definition: the experience of well-being due to harmonious mind-body integration. The orientation here is important, for health becomes an affirmation rather than an avoidance, a moving toward rather than a flight from. Within the "prana principle" rests an even higher definition of health and heightened experience of well-being. Here the focus is on prana, the inner-life force, and its potential to not only harmonize body and mind, but to guide us to its most subtle expression within us, that of "spirit". There is not only the affirmation of life, but the truest experience and celebration of our inherent potential for wholeness and "holiness". For if we follow the continuum of prana, we begin to experience the infinite, sublime seed of life within us. Such an orientation to health holds profound implications for how we live our lives and the fundamental attitudes we hold toward it.

Where Do I Go From Here?

The first step on the Kripalu path to Holistic Health is to establish where you are now. The next section of this book is a specially developed Holistic Health Appraisal Checklist which will help you draw a base line from which you can measure your progress and your needs. By completing it before you read on, you will more strongly experience the benefits of the chapters that follow.

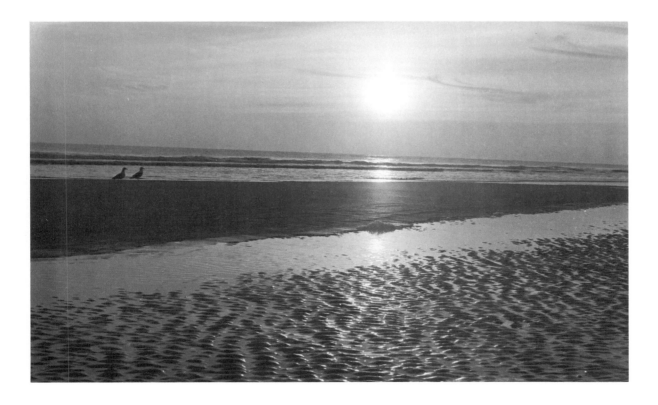

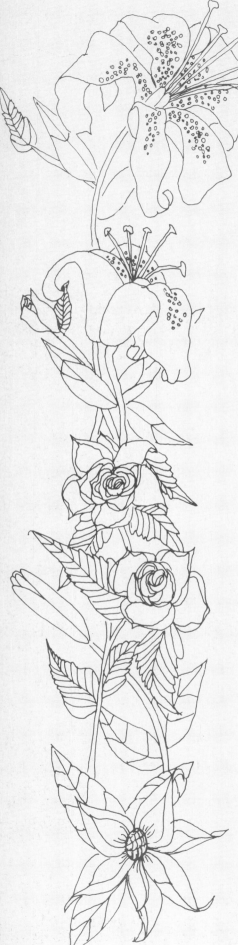

Self-Discovery

Check Out Your Holistic Health Quotient

The questionnaire which follows has two main purposes: (1) to provide you with insights into your current Holistic Health quotient, which will be a basis for understanding and practicing the methods suggested in this book; and (2) to be a baseline against which you can check your progress after you have implemented these techniques in your daily life for a period of time. It has been constructed in such a way that you can repeatedly complete it and record your score about every 3 to 6 months, seeing areas of improvement as you progress. NOTE: It is important to answer the questions objectively, recording what you really do, not what you would *like to think* you do! Circle the number which corresponds most closely to what you do.

% of time	80-100%	60-80%	40-60%	20-40%	0-20%
1. Relaxation					
a. I am generally relaxed and unworried.	5	4	3	2	1
b. I sleep well and regularly.	5	4	3	2	1
c. I fall asleep easily without help.	5	4	3	2	1
d. I have no trouble getting up.	5	4	3	2	1
e. I take a brief relaxation/meditation daily.	5	4	3	2	1
2. Body					
a. I feel fit, energetic and healthy.	5	4	3	2	1
b. I take responsibility for illness.	5	4	3	2	1
c. My body feels flexible and youthful.	5	4	3	2	1
e. My weight and muscle tone are good.	5	4	3	2	1
3. Exercise					
a. I do vigorous exercise (jog, tennis, etc.) often (3 or more times a week).	5	4	3	2	1
b. I do stretching, limbering and yoga daily.	5	4	3	2	1
c. I dance or express myself through my body.	5	4	3	2	1
d. I work ongoingly at improving my fitness.	5	4	3	2	1
e. I walk rather than drive whenever I can.	5	4	3	2	1
4. Leisure/Fun					
a. I have energy to use my free time creatively.	5	4	3	2	1
b. I feel free to simply have fun without a purpose.	5	4	3	2	1
c. I laugh freely and frequently.	5	4	3	2	1
d. It's easy for me to joke with others.	5	4	3	2	1
e. I don't take life too seriously.	5	4	3	2	1
5. Work					
a. I enjoy my work to the fullest.	5	4	3	2	1
b. I feel fulfilled and appreciated.	5	4	3	2	1
c. I work a moderate number of hours, avoiding excess overtime.	5	4	3	2	1
d. My communications with co-workers are open and harmonious.	5	4	3	2	1
e. I experience little anxiety, insecurity or competitiveness.	5	4	3	2	1
6. Diet					
a. I eat natural, wholesome foods without additives.	5	4	3	2	1
b. I avoid "junk" foods like soft drinks, chocolate bars, etc.	5	4	3	2	1
c. I eat knowing that food affects my consciousness.	5	4	3	2	1
d. I fast/follow a purification diet.	5	4	3	2	1
e. I avoid stimulants such as coffee, alcohol, colas, and cigarettes.	5	4	3	2	1
7. Communication/Self Expression					
a. I communicate easily and openly with others.	5	4	3	2	1
b. I am comfortable with new people and groups.	5	4	3	2	1
c. I am a good listener.	5	4	3	2	1
d. I feel free to ask when I need love or caring.	5	4	3	2	1
e. I deal well with my own and other people's emotions.	5	4	3	2	1

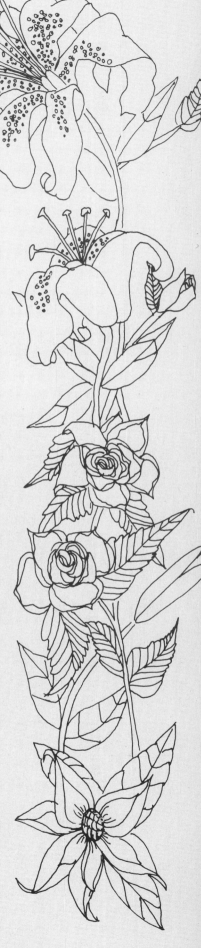

8. Spirituality/Meditation

	80-100%	60-80%	40-60%	20-40%	0-20%
a. Spirituality plays a role in my life.	5	4	3	2	1
b. I meditate or spend time in introspection.	5	4	3	2	1
c. I meet regularly with others for inspiration.	5	4	3	2	1
d. I express my spirituality in song and music.	5	4	3	2	1
e. I use prayer/affirmation as a healing tool.	5	4	3	2	1

9. Lifestyle/Environment

	80-100%	60-80%	40-60%	20-40%	0-20%
a. I feel that my lifestyle supports my health and spiritual needs.	5	4	3	2	1
b. The people I spend my time with are kindred spirits and help me grow.	5	4	3	2	1
c. I do everything in my power to foster my own health and well-being.	5	4	3	2	1
d. I am always seeking new ways to grow.	5	4	3	2	1
e. My family life is peaceful and harmonious.	5	4	3	2	1

Bonus Points

Now, simply pick the one statement that comes closest to describing your predominant feeling as you were filling out this questionnaire. Of course none of them will exactly describe your feelings, since you are unique, so just pick the one that is closest.

a. I expect I'll get a really high score, because I know I'm doing all I can. I can't wait to see the result. ( )

b. I'll probably score well in some areas and poorly in others, and that's OK. It'll be interesting and I'll learn about myself. ( )

c. I hope I'score well. I don't want to find out I'm not as healthy as I think I am. ( )

d. I don't suppose I'll score very well. I know I should be doing much more for myself. ( )

e. Oh dear, I bet I'll get a really low score and then I'll feel awful about myself. Perhaps I won't fill it out. ( )

How to Evaluate Your Score

There are two things to understand in evaluating your "score":

1. Only you can evaluate your "score". We are not going to give you a range of numbers and tell you a certain score is good or bad. This isn't like any other test you've ever taken because there is no pass mark, no norm against which to evaluate yourself, and no expectation for you to meet. The whole point of the quiz is for *you* to see yourself more clearly so you can decide what the implications are *for you personally.*

Then why are there numbers? So that you can use this quiz ongoingly to monitor your progress as you implement the methods outlined in the book. If you score yourself each time it is easier for you to see where you have made significant progress. The only important function of the numbers is for you to compare yourself to yourself over time -- say every three or six months.

Here are some suggestions for understanding the meaning of your first non-evaluative "score". Ask yourself:

Am I satisfied with what I see, in terms of overall results?

In terms of each individual section?

Does this tell me that I am as healthy as I can reasonably expect to be at this stage in my life?

Is my level of health and fitness normal for my age?

Do I want something more than health and fitness?

Am I doing the most that I reasonably can to nurture my health?

What more could I /would I like to do?

How much of a priority is this for me?

What stands in my way?

How can I use these answers to help me get more out of this book? Which areas am I strong in, and where do I have the potential for improvement?

2. Your attitude is more important than your score. The last question may have clued you in to this. It is more important to have a healthy, positive attitude to your health than to get a high score in this quiz. The questions were developed to help you to see where you are right now, and where you have the potential to improve. They were not developed to make you feel guilty for all the things you are not doing "right", or "should" be doing. In fact, if there were a score, we'd tell you to deduct at least 50 points if you felt guilty, self-rejecting or "bad" when you filled out the questionnaire! The best way to interpret your findings is with objectivity and lack of emotion, to the extent that you are able. It seems to be a natural human tendency to see our inadequacies more clearly than the things we are doing right. So look at your answers in this spirit: "Some things I'm doing right; some are areas that I haven't developed yet in myself. That's exciting because learning is always interesting, especially learning about myself. Who said I had to be perfect, anyway?"

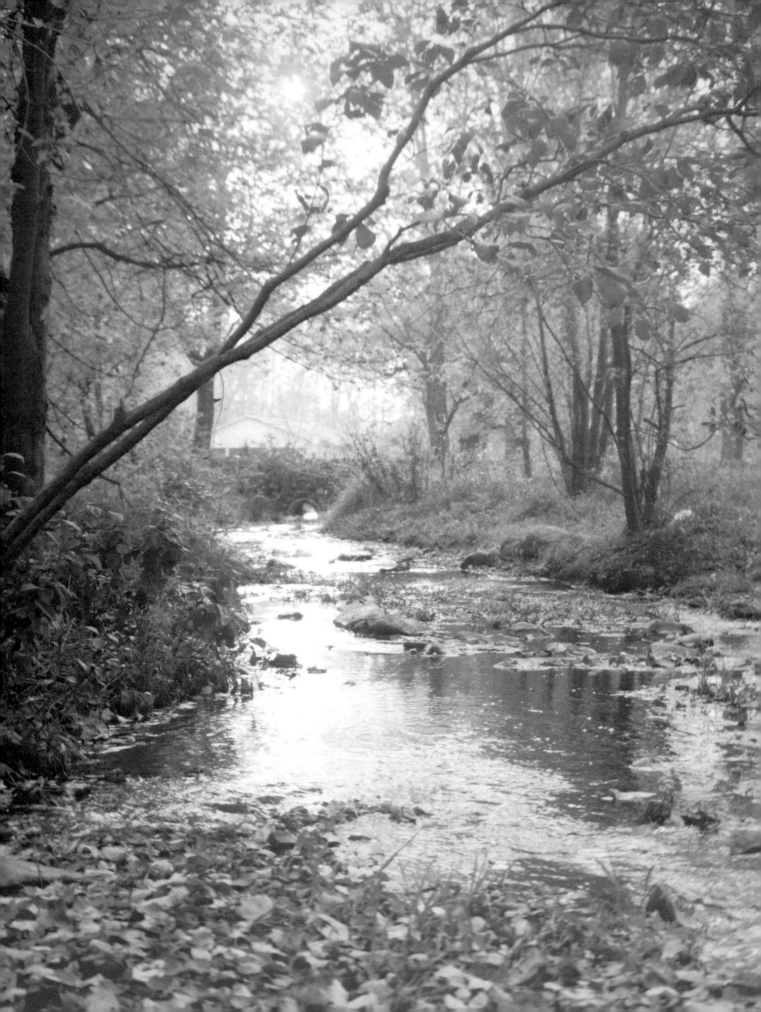

SECTION TWO

the answers: the Eightfold Way

INTRODUCING THE EIGHTFOLD WAY

The Kripalu Approach is a special combination of Holistic Health techniques from East and West. They have been tested over many years, most recently at the Kripalu Center for Holistic Health in Southeastern Pennsylvania.

The Kripalu Approach consists of eight simple pathways to health. They are based on the eight major ways that we express our energy in day-to-day living:

1. Living a More Relaxed Life
2. Getting to Know and Love Your Body
3. Learning How to Play
4. The Art of Relaxed Work
5. Discovering Your Own Optimum Diet
6. Communication & Self-Expression
7. Meditation and Spiritual Attunement
8. Creating a Supportive Lifestyle

These ways reflect what you might do in any 24-hour day to maintain your life's activities and relationships. In the Kripalu Approach each one plays a significant and equal role in life. Each one is a means through which you gain, lose, express and interact with the prana energy within you. The natural tools of Holistic Health -- borrowed from both modern and ancient traditions of healing, from massage to communications skills, from yoga to running -- provide ways to harmonize this energy in each area. Once you have created a total harmony of being, from how you eat to how you sleep, work or play, you naturally enter a realm of health beyond your present experience.

This approach to Holistic Health can be applied very practically. For example, guests at the Kripalu Center for Holistic Health practice living a daily schedule of yoga, relaxation, play, proper diet, etc., that gives them the opportunity to discover and establish positive health habits. Since there are varying degrees to which we are already in harmony with prana, most guests take a closer look at their health habits through the Health Appraisal, which indicates areas of imbalance. Practical tools are then learned that help establish a more harmonious lifestyle, one that is more supportive of their aspirations for perfect health. Once this has been properly understood, newcomers to Holistic Health soon realize what the French philosopher Peguy meant when he said that we die of how we've lived and we "live" of it too! Lifestyle is the keystone of Holistic Health.

It is our hope that this book will help you take your steps on the path to health easily with growing self-acceptance. This, in turn, will bring you the freedom and faith to grow and change.

Our present incomplete health and happiness are the result of choices we have made, consciously or unconsciously, throughout our lives. Now we are taking the responsibility to make new choices, to make changes. This requires energy and effort, but it is made easier if we accept the fact that habit patterns which took a lifetime to develop cannot be changed overnight. The ability to change while maintaining an attitude of flexibility and patience is essential. We must give ourselves permission to step forward and perhaps fall, to walk towards the sun of health, to take up a new habit, and occasionally to rest for a time in the shade of an old one. These qualities of self-acceptance, patience and sincerity are the hallmark of the healthy person. They will make it increasingly possible for you to use this book to walk towards health, nurturing the pleasure of your own company, your body, mind and spirit so that you experience the radiant energy of prana that is your birthright. The sun of health begins to rise in our hearts by one single significant step: that of looking. You've obviously already begun!

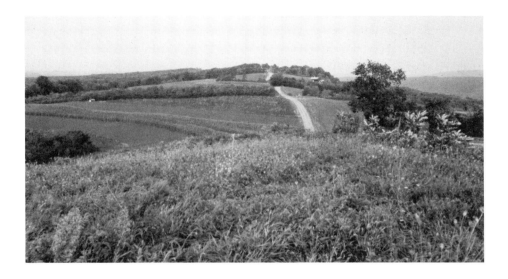

THE FOUR VOICES OF PRANA
by Yogi Amrit Desai

The Kripalu Approach to Holistic Health is based on becoming re-attuned to prana; that is, learning to live again in the most natural way possible, in accordance with the guidance of our inner life force, our prana. This inner energy empowers all the involuntary functions of the body harmoniously, creating and maintaining perfect health if we do not hinder it by becoming tense or ill. Prana can also be our guide in the areas over which we exercise conscious control. Unfortunately we have learned to live unnaturally over the centuries, not listening to this inner guidance. Instead, we make choices based on what we *think* we need, or simply on what will satisfy our five senses, rather than on what is good for the health of our bodies. Where once we were sensitive to the needs of our organism through intuitive knowledge of prana, we have lost even the capacity to hear those needs. We only hear our minds talking to us, not our bodies. Our goal is to re-establish communication with our prana; to learn to hear and heed its messages again.

One of the most basic levels at which we can re-establish our communication with prana is through the biological urges of the body. Prana communicates these life-giving messages to us privately and personally, sending them to the mind via the sensory nervous system. We can use this communication to re-establish our lost contact with the body and heighten our awareness of prana. Some examples of these messages are thirst (which is a signal that we need to drink liquids), fatigue (signaling a need to rest), hunger, tension, fullness of the bladder or colon, etc. All of these messages are actually a mild form of pain, so mild that we rarely think of them as such. Yet they are a form of pain and if they are attended to promptly and properly, they immediately turn to

the bliss of satisfaction and relief.

When we respond to these messages appropriately by promptly performing whatever action is indicated we reap increased physical health, vitality and mental peace. When we ignore, resist or postpone responding to prana's communication, prana's messages become more pronounced and urgent.

Prana communicates its signals to the mind in four stages of increasing intensity. In the first stage of communication prana attempts to draw the attention of the mind to the basic needs of the body. If this message is not heeded by the mind, prana escalates the intensity of its signals and, in the subsequent three stages, requests, insists and then demands the mind's cooperation in attending to the body's needs. Knowledge of these stages of prana's communication will make it easier for you to attune your mind to prana and to harmonize your daily activities to this inner wisdom. This will help you to become more holistically healthy and to avoid premature degeneration and aging of your body.

Stage One: Cooperation and Prevention

To insure the survival and sustenance of our body, prana needs our conscious cooperation. In stage one, prana signals the basic inner needs of our body to our mind through the sensory nervous system. These inner signals are experienced as urges to eat, drink, sleep, rest, or eliminate, etc. These needs must be met properly if prana is to efficiently fulfill its primary function of body maintenance, protection and healing. The function of the mind at this stage is to cooperate with prana by locating and securing from the external world whatever prana needs to sustain our body and keep it healthy. Whenever our mind cooperates and responds to these inner urges, it is functioning in harmony with prana and body.

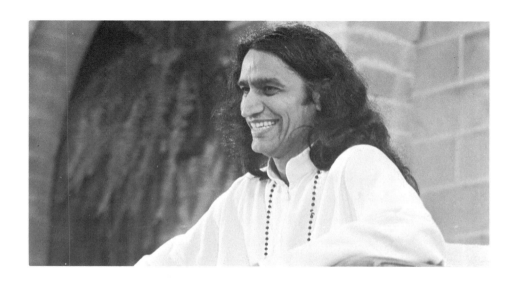

Thus, in contrast to the basic, involuntary state in which prana works independently of the mind's control, in this first stage prana is under the control of the mind. Here the mind has a choice: whether to follow prana's direction, ignore it, or resist or postpone responding to it. This is a crucial stage, where the mind can either choose to assist and support the sustaining, involuntary functions of the body by responding to prana's signals, or ignore these inner urges and disrupt the natural, involuntary functions of the body. For the mind to respond to the inner urges of the body and carry them out appropriately is an act of prana-mind or body-mind harmony. *This harmonious effort is preventive.* If the mind, however, turns its back on prana's signals and chooses to fulfill the ego's desires, dreams, fears and fantasies, it will automatically be in conflict with the body. Such conflicts of mind with the universal laws of prana, working through the body, lead to physical tension, mental restlessness, and strain, which are prana's way of signaling that we are straying from its guidance. If we do not change the orientation of our mind from the sensory desires of the ego back to prana we are eventually headed for trouble in the form of more serious physical and mental disorders.

Thus, during the first stage, the role of the mind is extremely important. Each of us has a choice to respond to the inner needs of our body as signaled by prana or to ignore these needs. Whether we respond to prana's signals by supporting the needs of the body or ignore prana's signals and postpone or resist fulfilling these needs is determined by the condition of our mind. If our mind is calm and clear, we will choose to fulfill the inner needs of the body. If the mind chooses to serve the ego's wants, it will choose a course of action that is not in tune with prana. For example, sometimes we respond to the needs of prana immediately, by resting when we are tired, by eating when we are hungry, by responding to the urge of elimination promptly, etc. By such

appropriate responses, we keep our energy high and insure good physical health. At other times, however, we may delay or resist responding to prana's signals and, as a result, our store of energy is depleted and our body suffers unnecessary wear and tear. Often we respond to the needs of prana only partially, such as by eating promptly when we are hungry, yet eating foods that emphasize taste rather than nourishment. Sometimes we ignore prana because of peer pressure, such as by staying late at a party we're not really interested in or following social customs such as wearing tight, constricting clothing in which we know our bodies are not comfortable. Sometimes we tune out the inner messages of prana and instead follow guidance which we get from outside ourselves which may not be suited to our individual needs, such as the latest health fads or diet theories.

Thus, at this stage, prana needs our conscious cooperation in fulfilling our body's needs and we have a choice: to respond to prana's signals or to ignore them. The first course of action is preventive and leads to physical health, mental peace and spiritual growth. The second course of action leads to physical discomfort and pain (Stage Two), acute bodily disorders (Stage Three), and eventually to critical, life-threatening bodily breakdowns (Stage Four).

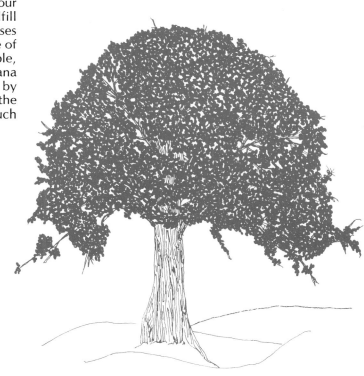

Stage Two: The Early Warning Signals of Sickness

In this stage, short-term pain prompts action, although there is still some choice. If our mind has ignored prana's signals and not responded to the needs of the body in Stage One, prana must correct the imbalance which we have created. Because the neglected need is causing increasing wear and tear on the body, prana is now forced to escalate the intensity of its messages to the mind in the form of greater pain, distress, tension or strain. The pain, at this stage, is only of sufficient intensity to become noticeable to the mind, which has successfully ignored the signals of the previous stage. For example, if we ignore prana's signal to empty our bladder when we get the first signal of slight discomfort, this discomfort eventually intensifies so much that we must pay attention to it. Or, as another example, if we postpone responding to prana's earlier signals of tiredness to quit working for the day, prana will increase the intensity of the message by signaling the need to rest with a headache, backache, fatigue, eyestrain or irritability. This is prana's method of getting our attention, letting us know that we are mistreating our body in some way. During this warning stage the messages from prana may be only occasional mild pain, fatigue, or minor physical disorders such as colds, indigestion, slightly elevated blood pressure, etc. Accompanying these physical complaints may be mental tension, irritability, and minor emotional disturbances. If we respond to these messages prana can correct the imbalance we have created in a short time, with a minimum of strain on our body. The occasional discomfort or pain is the price we must pay for ignoring the signals of the first stage and to restore the bodily imbalance we have created. If we ignore this pain or suppress it with tranquilizers, antacids, aspirin, etc., and continue to put excessive strain on our body, it will begin to deteriorate further.

At this stage we may be tempted to treat the symptoms in such a way as to achieve immediate relief from the symptoms, rather than going to the real cause of the problem. By allowing ourselves to ignore the first stage signal of prana we create a situation in which it is possible for us to misdirect our efforts toward a superficial or temporary solution to the immediate problem (the symptoms of increased pain) rather than to correct the true cause of the problem by responding to the original bodily need. This is the major difficulty of allowing ourselves to go beyond the first stage of prevention, in which we respond immediately to prana's signals. The earlier you respond to a bodily need, the less effort it takes to rectify the imbalance and the greater will be the results of your effort. Prevention is always better than cure.

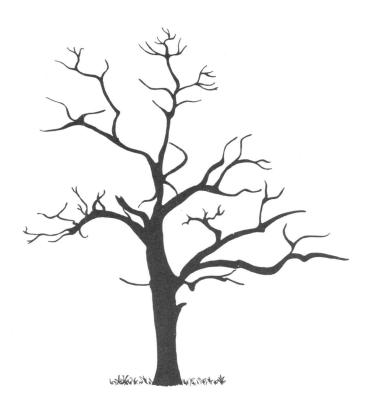

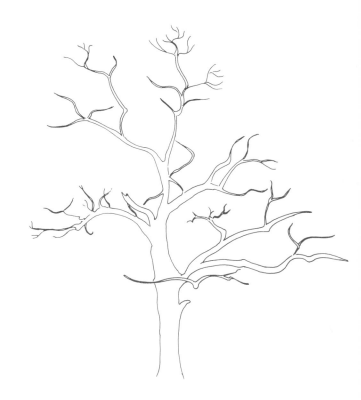

Stage Three: The Need for Cure

In this stage, fear of long-term pain and disability virtually forces us to act. If we fail to respond to prana's warnings as explained in Stage Two and continue to treat our body with the same lack of consciousness, prana must now resort to stronger, more obvious signals to draw the attention of our restless mind to the damage we are doing to our body. During this stage, prana sends signals of intense pain to warn us that various problems are now beginning to develop in our body. The more serious disorders and diseases which are now beginning to manifest in our body as pain are prana's cry for urgent attention. What was indigestion in stage two has now become the first signs of a peptic ulcer. Moderately high blood pressure has developed into the symptoms of cardiac insufficiency, angina pectoris or a mild heart attack. Morning stiffness in the joints has become the pains of arthritis. Our condition demands medical attention. The signals of prana during this stage are usually strong enough to force even those who are out of touch with their body into seeking medical aid. Our body is now incapacitated for significant periods of time and we become fearful over our state of health. We rarely have much energy, for prana is mainly occupied with constantly repairing the accumu-lated damage as well as the damage we are continuing to inflict upon our body. This state of low energy makes us less efficient at our day-to-day responsibilities. Our inefficiency makes us tense and, as a result, we become even less efficient and more fearful. This becomes a constant drain on our physical, mental, emotional and financial resources, and we may begin to develop psychological problems such as chronic anxiety or depression. For treatment to be successful at this stage we must seek professional assistance, change our lifestyle and practice attending to our bodily needs. Thus, we must attend to that which we ignored in Stage One, but with more pain, more effort, and less effectiveness. If these two regimens -- external and internal change -- are not followed conscientiously and wholeheartedly, our physical condition will deteriorate into Stage Four.

Stage Four: Incapacitating and Life-Threatening

In this stage fear of death controls our actions and we have no choice whether to respond or not. If we have not changed our lifestyle as indicated in Stage Three and have continued to overstrain our body, the condition of our affected bodily organs

MIND & PRANA -- A TRAGI-COMEDY IN PICTURES

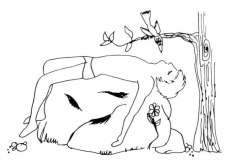

In the beginning, the body was limp and lifeless until....

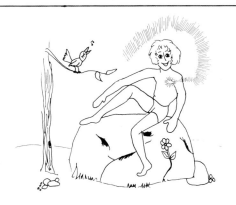

Prana, the life force, joined the body and gave it life!

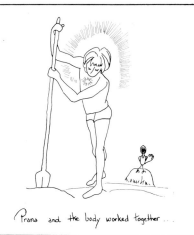

Prana and the body worked together....

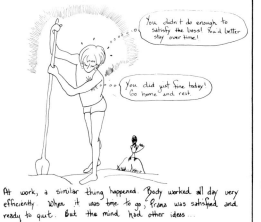

At work, a similar thing happened. Body worked all day very efficiently. When it was time to go, Prana was satisfied and ready to quit. But the mind had other ideas....

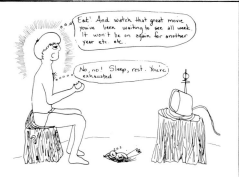

After pushing into overtime at work, the body is exhausted. After being ignored all day, prana's voice is weaker and makes very little impression on the mind.

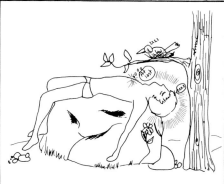

Body, now totally out of touch with the voice of prana, collapses.

and systems will continue to deteriorate. Prana now steps up the intensity of its signals to Stage Four. In this stage self-cure is almost impossible and we experience a critical breakdown of organs or systems in our body, requiring immediate, often radical, medical intervention in the form of hospitalization, major surgery, intensive care and prolonged convalescence. Often there is long-term physical disability which can make it difficult or impossible for us to provide for our own needs or continue to support a family. Some of the physiological and psychological conditions that are typical of Stage Four are: stroke with partial paralysis, perforated ulcer necessitating removal of part of the digestive system, acute psychosis or suicidal depression requiring hospitalization, massive heart attack, cancer, etc. In this stage prana's ability to work freely to accomplish healing is so inhibited by the physical and emotional blocks we have accumulated, from ignoring prana's signals in previous stages, that it can't recover easily to heal the body or mind's condition. It is barely able to drive the most vital organs and systems to keep the body clinically alive.

Only when the mind has failed to accept -- because of its preoccupations, conditioning and distractions -- all the accumulated violations of prana in the previous stages does prana resort to the intensity of its signals in Stage Four, which dramatically and urgently present to the mind the necessity of paying attention to the body if the body is to survive. Thus, prana upgrades the intensity of its signals in each successive stage only enough to capture the attention of the mind, and no more.

All stages of physical distress, from mere discomfort through severe pain, are simply messengers of prana with a single, simple purpose: to show us where we are going astray on the road of life and health, and to bring us back. They are like welcome lighthouses glimpsed through the fog, warning us to take our bearings and correct our course before we steer onto the rocks. Once we understand this, a change will happen in our attitude towards pain and sickness, health and life itself. We will become willing and able to respond to the warning signals that prana puts out in the earliest stage, and so lead a life of prevention rather than cure, a life that is full of the joy and freedom of Holistic Health.

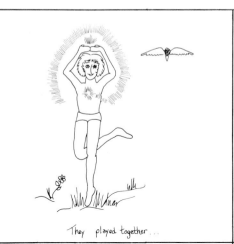

They played together...

Prana and the body worked together in perfect harmony. They listened to each other's needs very attentively. Whenever prana needed to eat, body ate. Whenever prana needed to sleep, body slept... Thus body and prana lived in harmony, complete in themselves, happy and healthy. Pure mind observed, enjoyed and supported the natural friendship of body and prana.

Then, one day, the mind discovered dreaming and scheming... wanting to be the boss... It had many desires to fill... So mind began to manipulate to receive the things it wanted, in the way it wanted.

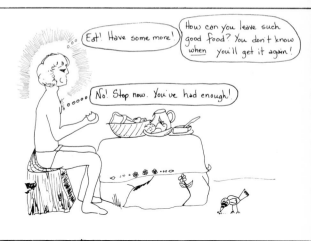

Eat! Have some more!

How can you leave such good food? You don't know when you'll get it again!

No! Stop now. You've had enough!

Many years pass....

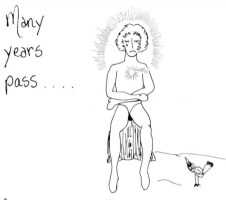

Body could hardly hear his friend prana anymore, which was pleading with him to stop, so ...

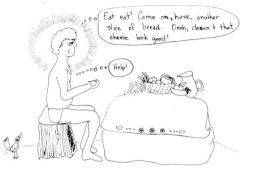

Eat eat! Come on, have another slice of bread. Oooh, doesn't that cheese look good!

Help!

After the body has been enslaved to the mind, he is in poor physical, mental and emotional shape... What can body do? One good look in the mirror says enough.

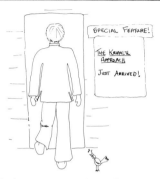

SPECIAL FEATURE!

THE KRIPALU APPROACH

JUST ARRIVED!

Yet body needn't despair. There is a way to return to that natural state of balance between the body and the mind....

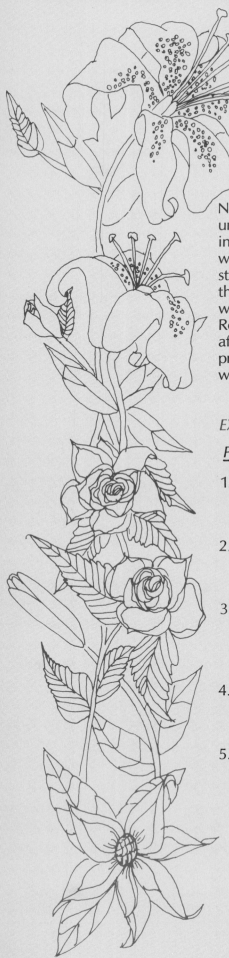

Self-Discovery

Test Your Ability to Listen to Prana

Now you can draw on your own experience for a more in-depth understanding of these principles. Find a quiet place to complete this introspection. Close your eyes for a moment and think of a situation where you felt conflicting urges. Below are some examples to get you started. As you get in touch with the situation, identify which voice was the voice of prana, of inner wisdom, of your real physical need, and which was the voice of the desires stimulated by your mind and senses. Remember what you did and then how you felt, physically and mentally, afterwards. Think of several such situations, some where you listened to prana and some where you listened to your mind. You may want to write them down to help you see a pattern.

EXAMPLE:

Prana said:	*Mind said:*
1. "Yawn! I need to go to bed."	"But I want to watch the Late, Late Show. It's especially good tonight."
2. "OK! I've eaten enough. I don't need any more."	"But this lasagne's so delicious. And who knows when I'll be able to have some again!"
3. "This room is so stuffy, and I'm stiff from sitting here all day. I need some fresh air and exercise."	"But I want to get this project finished so I'll get praise when the boss comes.
4. "Get up and go jogging; you'll feel great afterward."	"But I'm so warm and comfortable and sleepy. I must need the extra rest."
5. "You'd better not combine those two foods. You know they'll upset your digestion."	"It won't hurt just this once."

Experience 2

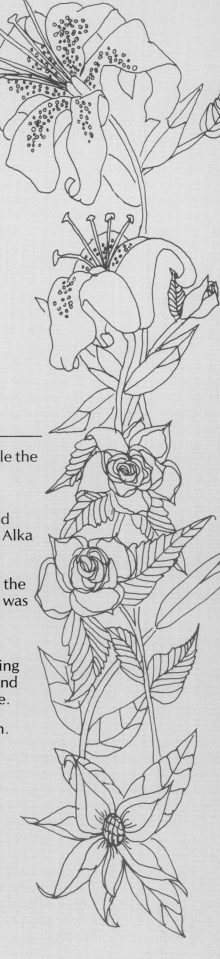

I did:

I stayed up.

I ate it.

I took a short, brisk walk.

I stayed in bed.

I saved one for later.

I felt:

I felt very tired and irritable the next day.

I felt too full, sluggish, and upset, and had to take an Alka Seltzer.

I felt revived and finished the project anyway because I was more alert.

I felt half-awake all morning because I slept too long and didn't get enough exercise.

I felt good, no indigestion.

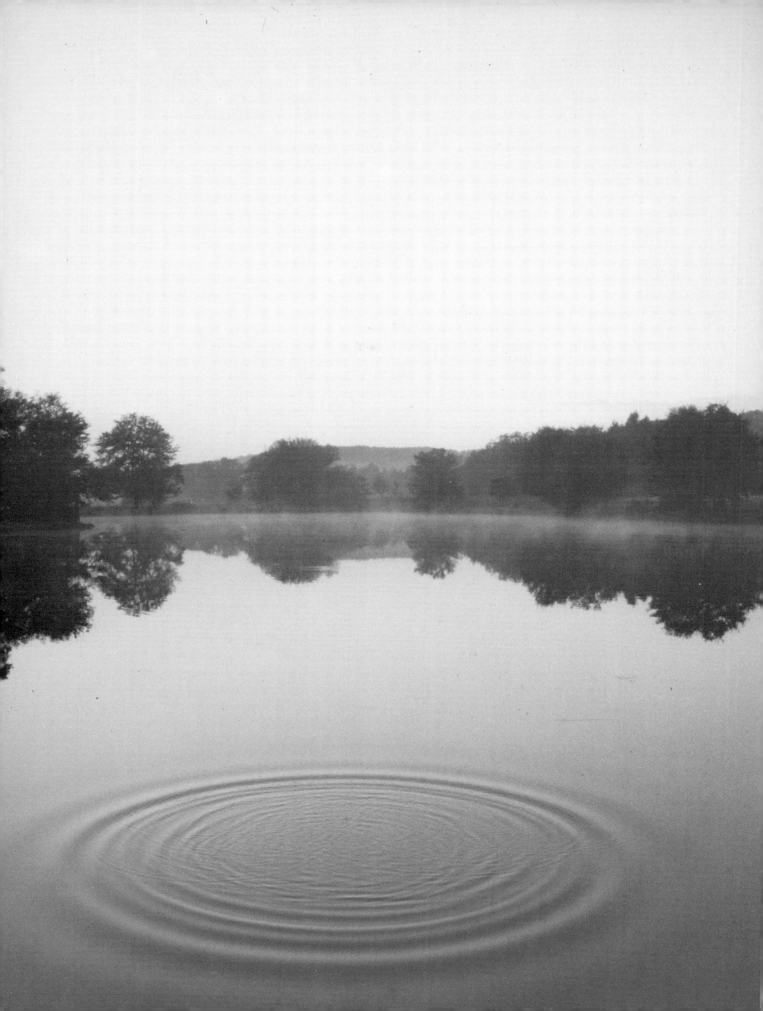

WAY ONE
living a relaxed life

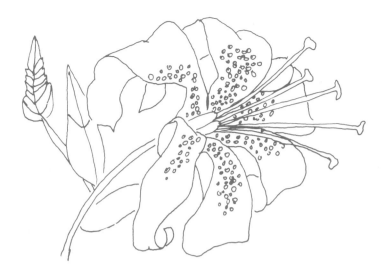

RELAXATION IS AN ATTITUDE

*Each time you feel tension it tells you that
there is something that needs your attention.
Tension is the result of our lifestyle, our past,
our expectations...it is the basic block
between us and the universal energy of
prana. When there is relaxation we become
like a sponge and draw energy from our
surroundings, whether we know it or not.*

In the active work-a-day world it's easy to
forget that rest and relaxation are as crucial to our
well-being as the air we breathe or the food we
eat. Throughout the night, as we dwell in the
deepest of relaxations, nature (prana) proceeds to
heal us while the mind remains quiet and the body
still. The same deep healing that happens during
relaxed sleep can occur in the wakeful state as
well. Currently, scientists are discovering that this
state of relaxation is a natural response of the
body which many of us seem to have lost touch
with amid the hurry of modern Western life.

The articles that follow present a detailed
practical understanding of stress, tension and
relaxation. They express a philosophy that has
two fundamental principles: one, that stress is not
necessarily bad and does not automatically lead to
the experience of tension; and two, that relaxation
is much more than what you need when you are
feeling tense or what you do when you are not
doing anything else. Relaxation, in the Kripalu
Approach, is an attitude to life which can be cultivated. It is a way of living, a state to be
experienced in each moment, no matter what you
may be doing. If you can learn to live this way,
you will prevent, or greatly diminish, the accumu-
lation of tension which has been proven to cause
most of our prevalent diseases. The chapter also
includes some easy-to-follow exercises which will
help you to identify what causes you, personally,
to experience tension, whether mental or physical, and how to go about relaxing those specific
tensions.

Redefining Stress

"Stress" -- what does this word evoke for you?
Pressure, fearful situations, difficulty in relationships, accident and injury, demands and expectations, feeling inadequate -- these are some
responses that came to people's minds when they
were asked this question. What would you add to
that list? Interestingly, these are all negative (i.e.,
undesirable) situations and connotations. Yet the
world's foremost stress researcher, Dr. Hans Selye
of Montreal, defines stress as a purely neutral
physiological phenomenon, devoid of any value
connotations of desirable or undesirable. In his
view, stress is a "non-specific response of the body
to any demand made on it."* Only later, after we
have experienced the initial physiological reaction
to the external situation, does our conscious mind
interpret the experience as positive or negative.
Our association of the word stress with only undesirable phenomena is thus a one-sided definition.

Consequently, the first thing to understand
about stress is that it is a neutral, natural and
normal response of the body to any external situation which places a demand on the body's energy
resources. That includes most life situations.
Pleasure, joy, happiness and excitement also elicit
the body's stress response, but since we do not see
them as undesirable and seek to avoid them, the
energy drain is less and we do not experience
these emotions as "stressful."

Stress is not only a normal reaction of the body,
but also one which is necessary to the maintenance of our lives. Responding to stress enables
us to take the actions necessary to keep ourselves
alive, free from danger, and evolving as a species.
How then has stress become such a negative
concept in present day society? Eighty percent of
illnesses are said to be caused by stress, and
"stress management", "deep relaxation", and
"tension-release" are sought after by everyone.
Why the tension headaches, the ulcers, the whole
range of stress-related ailments if stress is a neutral, normal, natural part of being alive?

It is because we have not consciously examined
and understood this ancient, instinctual physiological stress pattern. We have not realized that
we are responding to stress at the same instinctual
level as our ancestors. Their stress response was
appropriate to them: life was precarious and the
ones who survived to propagate the species (i.e.,
our ancestors) were those who were fastest,

*from Stress Without Distress

strongest and fiercest in the face of the life-threatening situations which occurred daily. When they sensed danger an instantaneous instinctual response mechanism was triggered to protect them. The autonomic (instinctual) nervous system signaled the body to release the hormone adrenalin into the blood stream and this provided instant energy to the heart, lungs and muscles to adapt and adjust the organism for "fight or flight."

Our bodies still respond with this same ancient mechanism which rushes to us intense energy for fight or flight. But our lives have changed. What we now need is a new way of channeling this adaptive energy towards cooperation and interaction with others. Instead, as we have evolved as a species and gained the power to interpret our sensory inputs through the thinking process, these interpretations of the events around us have been intermingled and confused with our instinctual unconscious reactions. We are trapped in a maladaptation to our present level of evolution; caught on the stairway between an ancient, outdated but still active instinctual reaction and uncompleted conscious transcendence of that instinctual pattern. As a result, we do not cope effectively with the stress and we experience tension. Thus we need to start our process of learning to relax by making an important distinction between "stress" and "tension." *Stress is a natural, physiological phenomena necessary to life. Tension is the unpleasant physical and mental repercussion we experience when we are not able to process our stress effectively.*

From Stress to Tension

How has stress become tension? First, it is a result of our unconsciously continued habit of perceiving unexpected external situations as threatening, when in reality they need not be. In present-day society, trust, cooperation and interaction should be the way of life. Yet jungle law still prevails in our minds -- "survival of the fittest" is our unconscious law of life. This is a mechanical, instinctive response, not one made from conscious choice after objective understanding of the situation. If we overhear criticism of a task we have performed, we often respond with fear and anger as if it is a threat to our very life, rather than as what it is -- simply an evaluation of a task we happened to do less well than was expected. It is not even a judgment of us as individuals, just of an action of ours -- one of many. Yet our "survival of the fittest" internal mechanical programing says, "Defend yourself, or you will lose!" So we experience fear, as if our very life were threatened! That is our first mistake.

The second step at which we unconsciously set ourselves up to experience tension is in our lack of awareness of our physiological processes. We do not realize that our unnecessary fears are then generating a potential chain of physiological reactions (adrenalin secretion -- causing a rush of energy to muscles and heart for fight or flight) until it is too late. Our heart is thumping, we feel restless energy, and we start to experience a need to express it through anger or through vigorously

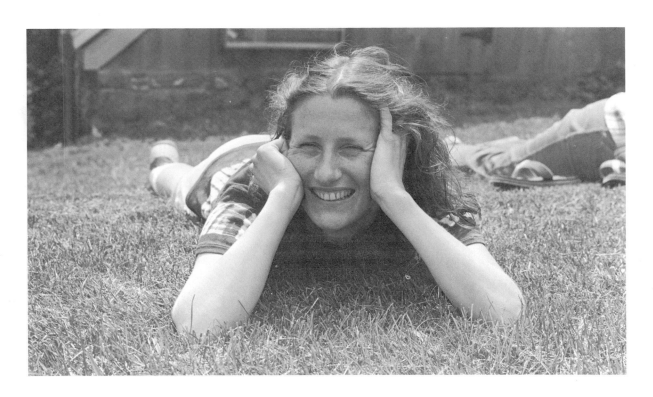

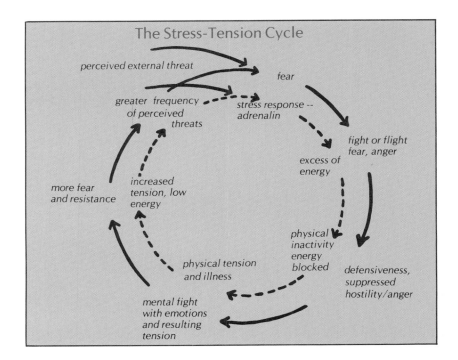

The Stress-Tension Cycle

perceived external threat

fear

greater frequency of perceived threats

stress response -- adrenalin

fight or flight fear, anger

excess of energy

more fear and resistance

increased tension, low energy

physical inactivity energy blocked

defensiveness, suppressed hostility/anger

physical tension and illness

mental fight with emotions and resulting tension

defending ourselves. Because the way we fight or flee is no longer physical but rather verbal, or even non-expressed, our bodies are full of excess energy released for intense physical activity. Because we do not consciously experience our negative emotions as simply energy coupled with inappropriate thinking patterns, we repress it as bad, antisocial, etc. This backed-up, unexpressed energy is then experienced as physical tension -- step three.

Another cause of tension is using mental energy to fight something we cannot physically control or change. For instance, if I am sitting in heavy traffic, not moving, and I know I am going to be late for an important meeting, I have two choices. I can fume and rage and be frustrated at the unplanned, uncontrollable and unnecessary delay. ("Why don't they do something about this bottleneck?" "Why don't people go home earlier, a different way?" "It's so stupid!") Or I can sit back, relax, and accept the inevitable. It's fairly clear that I will feel much more tense and drained by the first response than the second one, yet most of us respond in the first way.

We then do not like the feeling of accumulated tension and try to ignore it or release it in inappropriate ways (alcohol, drugs, sex). This non-acceptance of our basic physical-emotional experience is a further creator of tension. The tenser we become, the more we lose energy; the lower our energy, the more prone we are to perceive neutral events as threats, to experience fear, and to start the cycle over again. So tension is a downward spiral, fueled by fear and lack of conscious understanding.

Tension, then, is not inherent in a situation or caused by someone else. Although, at our present point in history, we are probably surrounded by more *potentially* tension-creating situations than ever before, we can learn to respond to these situations without tension. In fact our very survival as a species may depend on learning to do this since an estimated 80% of illness is believed now to be stress-related.

Evidence abounds for this all around us, but we have not seen it clearly. The same situation can "make" one person extremely tense, angry or fearful, while someone else is able to remain relatively relaxed and unconcerned. For instance, I may experience a visit to the dentist as extremely stressful and become very tense. You may remain completely relaxed and joke your way through the experience. We are all the end-products of different "programing" -- what evokes fear in one simply does not press another's panic button. And some of us simply have more fear programed into us in general. That's just the way it is. So what?

Two Ways to Break the Tension Cycle: Physical and Mental

What is the solution? How can we break the tension cycle and learn to be more relaxed, happy human beings? This is what the Kripalu Approach is all about. It teaches that we can intervene in the cycle at every stage in the process on two different levels: physical and mental. On the physical level, we can practice many different forms of bodily relaxation. This will raise and balance our energy (prana) which will render us less prone to experiencing events and people as threatening. We can learn to intervene in and override the physiological fight-or-flight response through special breathing exercises (two of these are detailed in the following chapter, Way Two) for breath is the link between mind, body and emotions.

On the mental level, we can intervene by accepting responsibility for our evolution as conscious beings and refusing to go on responding mechanically and instinctually as if every unexpected and undesired event is a potential threat to our survival. We can consciously observe our feelings of tension and trace them back to the fear or the imagined threat, seeing that it was not so, that it was merely a threat to our pride, or to our security, to our superficial ego. This means learning to re-interpret our world, to change the attitudes that we feel are a part of "us" and with which we feel secure (if unhappy)! A wise man has said, "We must, at every moment, be prepared to give up what we are for what we can become."

Living a relaxed life will begin to happen as we consciously develop a new adaptive process for dealing with the stresses in our lives. We can cultivate an alternative to the fight-or-flight polarization: acceptance of and cooperation with whatever situations life sends our way. As we flow with the current in the river of life we will be attuned to prana, which *is* that current. Tension will then diminish little by little until it becomes a thing of the past.

The exercises and articles that follow have been structured to help you become more familiar with how you personally convert stress into tension. They also provide many concrete, practical techniques both for overcoming your stress response in specific kinds of situations and for leading a more relaxed life in general.

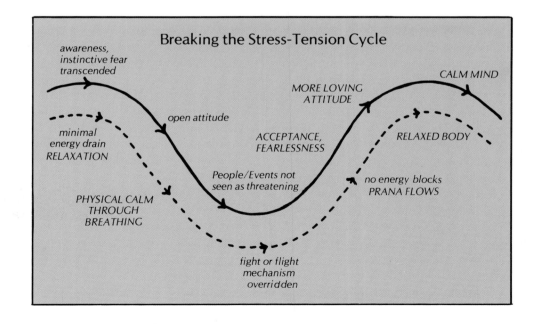

Breaking the Stress-Tension Cycle

awareness, instinctive fear transcended

minimal energy drain RELAXATION

open attitude

MORE LOVING ATTITUDE

CALM MIND

ACCEPTANCE, FEARLESSNESS

RELAXED BODY

People/Events not seen as threatening

PHYSICAL CALM THROUGH BREATHING

no energy blocks PRANA FLOWS

fight or flight mechanism overridden

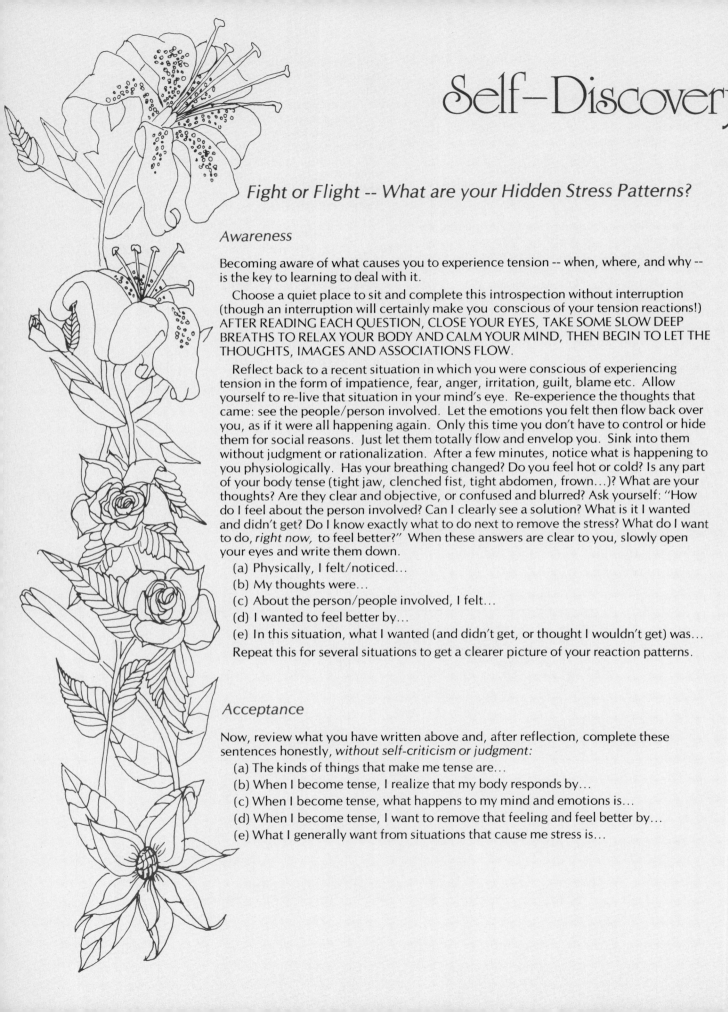

Self-Discovery

Fight or Flight -- What are your Hidden Stress Patterns?

Awareness

Becoming aware of what causes you to experience tension -- when, where, and why -- is the key to learning to deal with it.

Choose a quiet place to sit and complete this introspection without interruption (though an interruption will certainly make you conscious of your tension reactions!) AFTER READING EACH QUESTION, CLOSE YOUR EYES, TAKE SOME SLOW DEEP BREATHS TO RELAX YOUR BODY AND CALM YOUR MIND, THEN BEGIN TO LET THE THOUGHTS, IMAGES AND ASSOCIATIONS FLOW.

Reflect back to a recent situation in which you were conscious of experiencing tension in the form of impatience, fear, anger, irritation, guilt, blame etc. Allow yourself to re-live that situation in your mind's eye. Re-experience the thoughts that came: see the people/person involved. Let the emotions you felt then flow back over you, as if it were all happening again. Only this time you don't have to control or hide them for social reasons. Just let them totally flow and envelop you. Sink into them without judgment or rationalization. After a few minutes, notice what is happening to you physiologically. Has your breathing changed? Do you feel hot or cold? Is any part of your body tense (tight jaw, clenched fist, tight abdomen, frown…)? What are your thoughts? Are they clear and objective, or confused and blurred? Ask yourself: "How do I feel about the person involved? Can I clearly see a solution? What is it I wanted and didn't get? Do I know exactly what to do next to remove the stress? What do I want to do, *right now,* to feel better?" When these answers are clear to you, slowly open your eyes and write them down.

    (a) Physically, I felt/noticed…

    (b) My thoughts were…

    (c) About the person/people involved, I felt…

    (d) I wanted to feel better by…

    (e) In this situation, what I wanted (and didn't get, or thought I wouldn't get) was…

Repeat this for several situations to get a clearer picture of your reaction patterns.

Acceptance

Now, review what you have written above and, after reflection, complete these sentences honestly, *without self-criticism or judgment:*

    (a) The kinds of things that make me tense are…

    (b) When I become tense, I realize that my body responds by…

    (c) When I become tense, what happens to my mind and emotions is…

    (d) When I become tense, I want to remove that feeling and feel better by…

    (e) What I generally want from situations that cause me stress is…

Experience 3

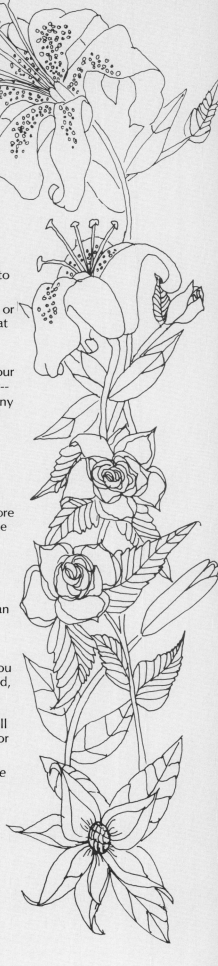

Adjustment

How to Transform Your Tension Reaction into a Relaxation Response

Now that you understand more clearly how your tensions are caused, you can begin to find ways to relax in those situations.

1. *Begin to observe yourself* ongoingly and see tension approaching from a distance, or catch it happening. Then accept it! If you fight it and try to suppress it, or get angry at yourself for reacting in that way, you'll get more tense, lose more energy. Just recognize it and allow yourself to feel the symptoms in your body.

2. *As it happens, begin to consciously relax* by breathing more slowly and deeply. Your emotions are intimately connected to your breathing patterns (see "The Second Way-- Breathing") and so, by changing your breathing, you will quickly be able to change any chain of thought, even a stressful one. This, in turn, changes the physical responses that go along with emotional or mental tension, such as tightness in the abdomen, shoulders, etc. The beauty of it is that deep breathing can be practiced anywhere without anyone even noticing -- at work, while traveling, or in a situation of confrontation. So when you feel your body beginning to experience the tension response, immediately begin to take long, deep regular breaths. The natural way to breathe when relaxed is deeply and steadily (watch a sleeping child, or an animal at rest). As you breathe more deeply you will feel refreshed because you will take in more prana. You will feel more calm and objective, so that you will be able to deal with the situation itself more efficiently.

3. *Recognize* whether you are experiencing a fight response or a flight response, and see if you can *change your thinking/attitude* about the situation (See following exercises).

4. *Recognize* what you want from the situation and are not getting, and see if you can drop that wanting. Accept what is actually happening, rather than trying to fight mentally and emotionally for what you want to have happen.

5. *Examine* your daily routine to see if you are creating physical reasons which pre- dispose you to experience tension. You will be more likely to experience tension if you are over-tired from lack of sleep; if you have overeaten, eaten the wrong kinds of food, or eaten too late at night; if you have taken in too many stimulants (coffee, alcohol, cigarettes, etc.); if you overwork; if you don't get enough play and recreation; if you don't get enough fresh air and exercise, etc. See where you can make changes -- small ones, one at a time. Don't take on too much! Just regulate your sleep, for instance, or walk instead of driving once in a while to get more fresh air and exercise.

6. *Incorporate some specific physical and mental techniques into your daily schedule such as:* Hatha Yoga, running, meditation and sports. Also take time out to lie down and relax deeply, once a day, for 15-20 minutes.

TENSION IS AN ENERGY CRISIS
by Yogi Amrit Desai

Tension is an energy crisis. It arises from the misuse or abuse of energy. Tension is inefficiency; it is the inability to work at peak performance level. When a car is finely tuned all of the engine's moving parts work in total harmony with each other. As a result, that car gets the highest possible mileage with the minimum of gasoline. In other words, the output of energy is maximum. In the same way, each aspect of a person must work in harmony with all other aspects. The body must be healthy, the emotions balanced, and the mind attuned to the body, emotions and prana. Then our capacity to put forth effort and accomplish work is so high that we get the maximum amount of work done with the minimum expenditure of energy. This harmony of being is the true state of relaxation.

Seeking Harmony of Being

To create the state of total harmony of being, we must first know what creates the disharmony, the tension within us. Tension has two sources: physical disharmony and mental disharmony. Insufficient sleep, insufficient exercise, not eating or digesting properly -- these and other unbalanced physical habits can result in physical tension. Something as simple as posture can be a cause of tension. If we carry our bodies improperly, if we sit, stand or walk incorrectly, our bodies will be filled with tension. Each physical habit needs to be taken into consideration in order to effect a permanent change in our ability to relax.

Although tension can have definite physical causes, our mental attitude toward ourselves and our surroundings is the primary source of our disharmony and tension. For example, two of the chief causes of tension are competition and jealousy. When people are motivated to work by competition or jealousy, their purpose is defeated. Instead of gaining from their labor, they lose consistently, because competition and jealousy inevitably lead to fear and insecurity. Fear and insecurity give birth to tremendous tension as they feel pressured to work more efficiently at a job they often dislike. The need for efficiency gives birth to still greater tension as they begin to realize their own inadequacies. These feelings of inadequacy may manifest in either a superiority or an inferiority complex. These complexes prevent the people from understanding each other. Such misunderstandings create tension. Thus at every level of activity, they sink more deeply into an unending cycle of tension.

Living for Today

In order to escape the misunderstandings and feelings of inadequacy which arise in their external situation, these people then seek refuge in their imagination. They live in tomorrow, filled with hopes and desires for the future. The more they desire for the future, the less they are satisfied with today. Their increased dissatisfaction produces greater and greater tension. Thus their hopes for tomorrow cause greater incapacity to act efficiently today and they become increasingly more insecure.

To fight this self-produced insecurity, such people strive to pack more and more fun into their day, to consume more, to store more for tomorrow's fun. This striving creates more insecurity. The frantic fun-seeking, the need to collect and consume for tomorrow, brings many fears. People then have too many choices for today and too many desires for tomorrow. This makes them restless, insecure and incapable of enjoying life in the present.

Warning: Competition May Be Harmful To Your Health

This restlessness prevents such people from finding satisfaction, leading to dissatisfaction in their personal lives and dislike for their work. Dislike for work creates tension which further undermines their efficiency and leads to self-pity, lack of confidence and a destructive self-image. These feelings consume a tremendous amount of energy. Once depleted of energy, they suffer from depression, loneliness and fear. In order to forget their problems they may resort to drinking, smoking, overeating, excessive sex, drugs, and other forms of escape which either dull or artificially excite their nerves. To relax they often engage in the competition of the "game world." But even there they do not escape competition; they merely change the arena of competition because their competitive minds are still present. They try playing chess, or painting or golfing, but the game doesn't help them relax because they have not changed their competitive mental attitudes. So long as the newness of the sport lasts, they feel that they have changed.

Soon, however, the newness wears off. The habitual attitudes return, and recreation once again is just another source of aggression, fear, fighting, jealousy and tension. As a result they end up breaking their golf clubs on the golf course or tearing up their canvas in painting class. They cannot enjoy their work and they no longer know how to play.

If these people continue to resort to escapes and crutches, these escapes become subconscious drives and habits which bring the endless array of physical, mental and emotional disorders which result from the condition of stress: chronic fatigue, insomnia, restlessness, headaches, stomach ulcers, indigestion, constipation, obesity and pains in the back and shoulders. Tension creates all of these problems in the first place, but eventually each of these symptoms creates further tension, thus establishing a vicious cycle of tension.

Finding Inner Balance

The superficial changes to which the average person resorts provide only temporary solutions. The real answer to these problems is to go within and get in touch with one's true inner needs. While there has been astonishing progress made in the material world, most people have failed to adjust their inner lives to keep pace with their mounting external progress and prosperity. As a result, external progress and prosperity have become a burden rather than an asset to peace of mind. Through the practice of listening to prana, we learn the secrets of balancing body, mind and inner energies to function effectively amid the pressures of progress and prosperity in modern society. We learn to hear our inner requests for self-care and nurturance. Upon hearing them, if we choose to respond, we relieve ourselves of the tension of acting against our natural needs. We act in harmony with the inner forces of nature, of prana, which are always working to establish homeostasis -- a balanced, relaxed state of being. Prana is the whole secret of eliminating tension from our lives.

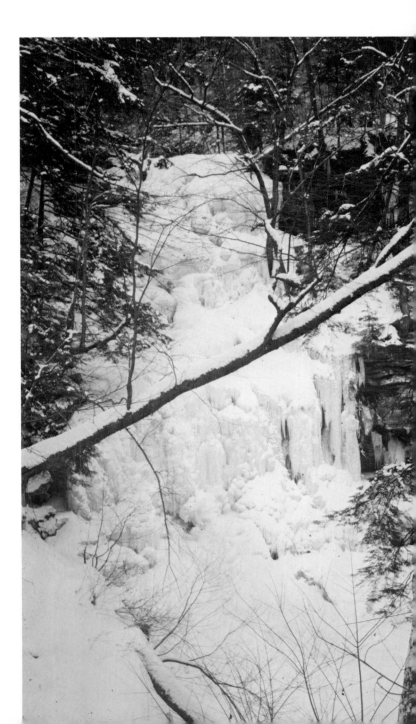

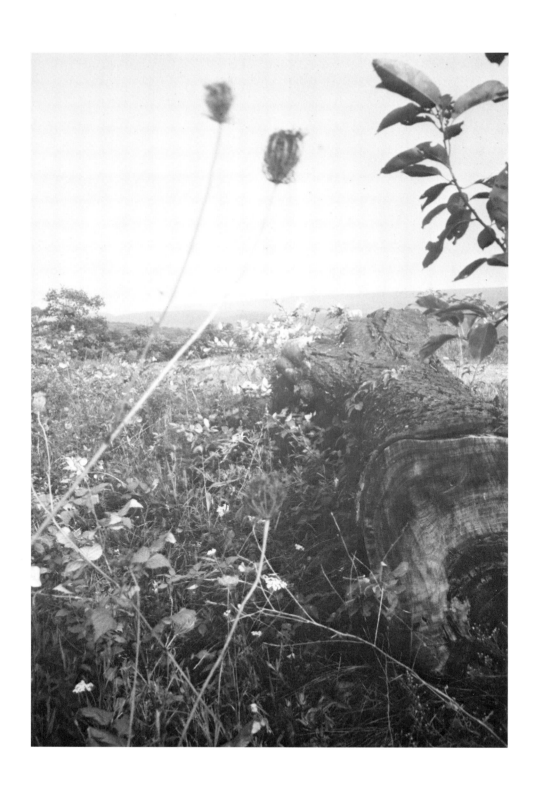

Self—Discovery Experience 4

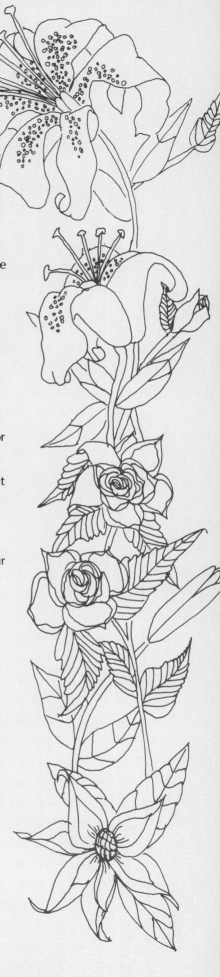

HOW TO REMOVE TENSION BY CHANGING YOUR POINT OF VIEW

Since most of our apparent problems simply come from lack of understanding, we can actually dissolve the tension they bring by changing the way we look at them. Resistance to stress -- that is, non-acceptance of the inevitable or what is presently happening -- causes most tension. We can remove this resistance by a better understanding of our attitudes. We can transform our "stressors" by changing how we view them. Use this introspection guide to help you pinpoint some attitudes that cause you unnecessary tension and see how to change them. Close your eyes and sit quietly before writing your answers to each question.

AWARENESS

1. Write down the names of some people to whom you characteristically react with a feeling of tension. Then write why it is that you think you have this reaction. In what way would you like the individuals concerned to be different than they are?

2. Choose a specific situation in the recent past that you remember as particularly stressful. What were the elements in that situation that caused you to react with tension and to experience unpleasant emotions? How would you have liked the situation to be different?

3. Look back at what you wrote in your first answer. Now see if you can write down, for each person, three of his or her good points and three useful things that you have learned about yourself from your interactions with them.

4. Look over what you wrote about the "stressful" situation. Reflect on it for a moment with your eyes closed. Then write down what you *now* see, with the perspective of time, that you learned from that situation. Write the main lesson in it for you, and then as many other learnings as you can.

ACCEPTANCE

1. Review all your answers. Now write down what you see about the way in which your attitude (your perspective, your point of view) affects your reaction to so-called stressful situations. How much stress is inherent in the situation and how much is caused by your own reaction to the situation, your ongoing point of view?

ADJUSTMENT

1. How will you handle these kinds of situations the next time they arise? Write down some *specific ways* in which you can *think differently,* and so reduce the amount of tension you experience in such situations.

2. Are you feeling self-rejecting or "bad" about what you discovered? This too is an unproductive way of thinking that causes tension, both in you and those around you! What you feel is what you project to others and how they, in turn, will feel about you. It is important, therefore, to think positively about yourself -- to love yourself for your good qualities, particularly your willingness to see your weak areas and work on them. So to help in this positive thinking about yourself:

3. List 10 qualities about yourself that you and/or other people appreciate.

4. Finally, list 10 things you're grateful for in your life. (If at the end of every day, you listed 10 things, or even five, that you were grateful for, you would be amazed at the change in your thinking patterns, particularly in the way you feel at the end of a so-called "bad" day.)

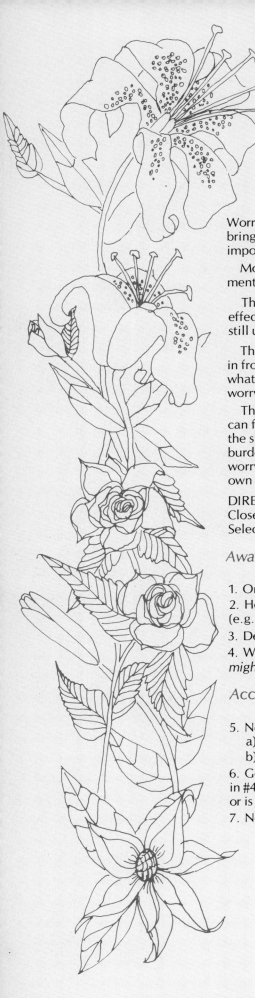

Self–Discovery

How to Stop Worrying in Nine Easy Stages

Worry is another energy drainer. It blocks the flow of prana, and sometimes even brings our mind and body to a standstill where constructive thought or action seem impossible.

More often than not, worry itself comes from our own vague and often distorted mental projection of the outcome of a situation, rather than from the situation itself.

This situation could be one that has already occurred in the past but may have effects in the present or future, or a situation of the present or future whose outcome is still undetermined. Worry and "the unknown" often seem to be companions.

The key to dealing with worry is to "demystify" it -- to set the elements of your worry in front of you for examination, separate the facts from the feared fantasy, and gauge what steps need to be taken for realistic decision-making and action. Action dissolves worry, which is nothing other than indecision or perceived inability to act.

The exercise which follows will assist you in the process of dissecting a worry so you can fearlessly examine its parts. You will find that choosing to take hold of a worry by the simple act of looking at it can be your first step toward relieving yourself of its burden and restoring your view to one of optimism and objectivity. Oftentimes, once worry has been dispelled, the eye of intuition opens and from within the depths of your own prana, your inner energy, an answer emerges that feels very clear and quite right.

DIRECTIONS: Sit down quietly in a secluded place where you will not be disturbed. Close your eyes for a few moments, breathe deeply and slowly, and relax. Then begin. Select a situation about which you are worried.

Awareness

1. On a sheet of paper, briefly describe the situation.
2. How often and how long have you worried about this? When do you worry about it (e.g. at meals, bedtime, on your break)?
3. Describe what happens to you, physically and mentally, when you worry about this.
4. What specifically do you imagine might happen? (Elaborate. Write *all* that you fear *might* happen.)

Acceptance

5. Now what is the *worst* that could happen?
   a) in the situation?
   b) to you?
6. Go back and re-read all that you've written. Especially examine what you've listed in #4 and #5. Take each point and consider: "Realistically, might this actually occur, or is it simply my mind fantasizing the worst?"
7. Now consider, if #4 and #5 did occur, is it "that bad"? Is all really lost?

Experience 5

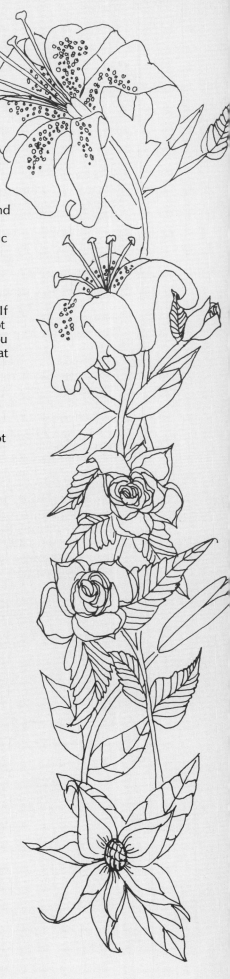

Adjustment

8. Again, consider what you've listed in #4 and #5. Take each point, *one at a time,* and determine if there are concrete steps you can take *now* to set the situation in order. For example: "I am worried the roof might cave in." After determining if this is realistic (you tested the beams and there's actual evidence) ask: "What concrete steps can I take?" Then list all the choices. In the case of the roof, you could: move out, call the landlord, put up new beams, etc.

9. Where possible, take these concrete steps to remove your worries. Where you see it is not possible, determine to simply drop your worrying and accept what happens. If you can't *do* anything about it, then at least determine to conserve your energy by not worrying. Not only does it not help (you knew that before) but it actually depletes you of physical and mental energy, so that you have less energy to deal with the things that you *can* do something about. Decide to be in the present, in the moment. Worry is living in the future -- uselessly. Take care of things the best way you can, and then surrender the rest to life. All the great masters have taught this profound truth. It's what Christ meant when he spoke of the birds of the air and the lilies of the field, and said "Which of you, by taking thought for the morrow can add one cubit to his stature?" He didn't mean that we should not be practical, or plan ahead; He meant not to waste our energy in continually thinking and worrying about the future! Be here now!

HOW TO PRACTICE YOGIC SLEEP-RELAXATION (YOGA NIDRA)

Like swimming, the true experience of deep relaxation can only be understood by jumping in and trying it. Follow the instructions below. Try to practice the technique regularly, at least once a day. Soon you'll become old friends with a state that is rightfully yours: the peace and tranquility of a tension-free body and mind. Such an experience will continue to be reflected in what you think, say and do. The experience will also help your ongoing awareness of your physical and mental states. You will come to recognize your potential for calm awareness, resiliency and adjustability to unexpected events or demands made upon you.

For many centuries yogis have used the technique of yogic sleep-relaxation as a highly effective method of recharging mind and body. You may feel that you are asleep, but in fact this exercise simply takes you to a different level of consciousness. This consciousness allows the inner intelligence of prana to move freely throughout your system, relaxing, rejuvenating and healing you on all levels -- mental, emotional and physical. Thus, by practicing it on a daily basis, you will gradually decrease the level of tension in all of your activities. Yogic sleep-relaxation may be done at any time. Remain in this state for a minimum of 15 minutes daily. As there is no set maximum time of practice, you may remain in yogic "sleep" for as long as your schedule permits. At first, you may find it easier to have a close friend quietly read you these instructions, until you have practiced and memorized them. You may also wish to send for one of our guided relaxation tapes (see appendix).

1. *Prepare your room, your family, yourself.* If possible, darken the room, see that the temperature will be comfortable for you (fairly warm, because the body will feel cool due to slower metabolism, as in sleep). Let your family members or co-workers know that you'd like twenty minutes by yourself. Close the door (perhaps lock it or put up a sign, so you will really feel secure from interruption) and begin to feel that this time is just for you. Lie down on your back and close your eyes.

2. *Regulate your breath.* Begin to take long, deep and uniform breaths, gradually slowing down the rate of your breath. By slowing your breathing tempo to the rate of approximately three heartbeats to each inhalation, five to each exhalation; your body and mind will also begin to relax and slow down. Continue with this breathing throughout each step until you completely lose awareness of it by having sunk deeply into relaxation.

3. *Progressively relax each muscle.* As you continue with deep breathing, begin to consciously relax your muscles. Mentally traveling over your body, tell each part to relax, one by one, from the toes to the top of your head. With each exhalation feel as if you are letting go, breathing out tiredness, stress, tension from that body part. With each inhalation, feel yourself breathing in relaxation.

Relax in this order: your feet, ankles, calves, knees, thighs, hips, abdominal muscles, the muscles of the back, chest, shoulders, arms and hands. Relax your neck and skull. Then relax your face. Drop any tensions which surround the eyes, and let all facial expressions fall away. Relax your forehead, and the sides of your face. Allow your jaw to sag slightly, parting your lips, and relax your tongue.

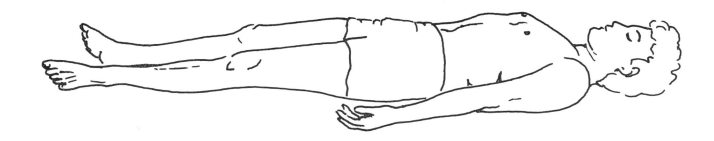

4. Relax each organ. Now bring your attention within your body to the internal organs. Without trying to guess their exact location, picture the organs of the abdomen: kidneys, liver, adrenal glands, stomach, intestines, bladder and reproductive organs. As you relax each organ, picture the deep tensions and organic disorders within dissolving at your mental suggestion to relax. Picture your lungs and heart. Feel their pace become slower, more even, free of disturbance or tension. Visualize your brain and imagine that the steady rhythm of breath is cleaning it of all tension -- dissolving thoughts, soothing and restoring the millions of cells that lie within it.

5. Calm your nervous system. When your muscles and organs have become relaxed, begin to consciously relax your nerves. Try to discover where the inner pockets of tension lie within your body. As they reveal themselves to your inner gaze, mentally visualize the incoming breath dissolving these buried tensions. Expel their last vestiges with your exhalation. Feel that your tired and overworked nervous channels are closing down, that communication between your brain and nerve centers is being temporarily suspended. Feel that you have completely let go, that your mind is like a clear blue sky with the thoughts as slowly floating clouds. Feel your body growing heavier and heavier as it sinks into the floor.

6. Calm your mind; let go. Now send your mind as far as it can go from your everyday life. Leave your anxieties and worries, your obligations and responsibilities. Create a strong mental image of a place where you are completely free, completely at peace. Perhaps you will visualize a sunny beach or a silent garden. Retreat into this, your personal sanctuary, leaving only your body lying on the floor. Be completely in your imagined retreat, in a state devoid of all fears for the future and all regrets over the past. Secure in the knowledge that you are at home within yourself, allow your conscious mind to drift into a state of blankness -- that state in which the inner intelligence of prana works to thoroughly heal and restore your being on all levels.

7. Gently come back. Stay in this state for as long as you wish. When your consciousness begins to return to your body, do not sit up right away. Instead, linger in the twilight state for a short time, gently stretching your body in the way that feels most natural for you. After a few minutes open your eyes and slowly sit up.

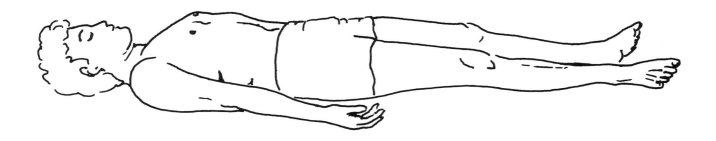

In Summary: Relaxation is a Way of Life

Relaxation is the result of doing many good things for yourself in your life, little as well as big, from proper diet to a positive attitude in your work. Remember that it comes from bringing about both physical and mental harmony in your life. After working with the physical approaches to de-stressing, you will have a keen awareness and energy to to enable you to look at the more subtle causes of tension: desires, likes, dislikes, expectations you may have of yourself or others, or that others may have of you. Working on this level of de-stressing takes an ounce more awareness and honesty, a pound more acceptance and patience. Allow yourself to experience self-esteem through your willingness to look, discover, change and grow.

Aspire to do good things in your life: 1) accept others through understanding rather than resisting or expecting that they'll change; 2) find one aspect of your work that you like and enjoy it thoroughly, performing it eagerly, and you will begin to gather energy to accept the less inspiring aspects in your work; 3) learn to look upon an unexpected change in events as an opportunity to acquire inner flexibility; 4) take the time to acknowledge the big and small things for which you can feel grateful, starting with a list of five each night, and soon your two hands won't be enough to count all your blessings; 5) and lastly, look upon yourself and others with patience, trust and love, remembering that we all create our life experiences by our own attitudes. Decide that yours will be a more relaxed attitude to life from now on.

OTHER RELAXATION TOOLS

Biofeedback has come a long way in the last ten years, from esoteric laboratory research technique to popular holistic health care tool. The word "biofeedback" simply means feedback from the body, but numbers of different machines have been developed to provide this feedback in varying ways. Each machine has essentially the same two functions: to read the body's internal signals of nervous activity and to amplify these signals and present them to their owner in visual or audible fashion so that he or she can learn to regulate them. Biofeedback is thus using modern technology to help us do what the sages of the East have been able to do for many centuries: to regulate the processes in our bodies that we have hitherto regarded as unregulatable, the processes of the so-called involuntary nervous system. Yogis have, for thousands of years, been able to control their heart beat, pulse, breathing rate, etc., but for the West this new knowledge is startling and even revolutionary.

Biofeedback

What are the implications of biofeedback for you, the reader interested in Holistic Health? Simply this. If you suffer from any form of physical tension, biofeedback is a useful tool for learning how to relax that tension. It is already widely used as a treatment modality for people who suffer from migraine headaches, for instance. By learning to increase the heat in their hands, they draw extra blood there, reducing the congestion in the blood vessels of the brain that seems to be the cause of migraines. In Kripalu terms, what biofeedback is really doing is reading the subtle signals of prana and relaying them to you. As you

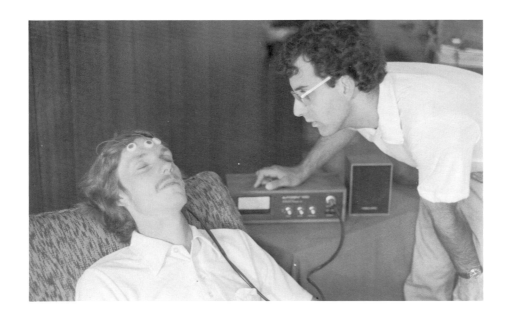

become more skilled at reading these signals for yourself and at spontaneously bringing relaxation to the different parts of your body, the need for a machine to act as intermediary will be transcended. This, of course, is the ultimate purpose of the Kripalu Approach. But we have found the use of biofeedback apparatus to be very helpful at starting people on the road to self-regulation and relaxation, and for monitoring their progress. If you have access to biofeedback training in your area, you will find it a rewarding way to begin to get in touch with your prana. To sit and watch a needle on a machine vacillating with every least twitch of your muscles, even with the thoughts that pass through your mind, is fascinating. Try thinking of a situation that makes you really angry, and see how the machine responds!

Note: There are a number of different kinds of machines on the market to read different manifestations of tension and bodily activity. The most popularly known reads the alpha (and other) waves of the brain. There are also the Electromyograph which reads muscle tension, primarily in the forehead, and GSR machines that read galvanic skin response. We have the latter two kinds at Kripalu Center for Holistic Health. Some are even small and inexpensive enough that you can buy them to use at home.

Hot Tub Therapy

Hot tubs are becoming so well-known that it is probably unnecessary to write about them. One of our most popular attractions at the Health Center is a large redwood hot tub. We recommend that you try the experience if one is available in your area.

The hot tub is an extremely relaxing and rejuvenating experience. Small, powerful jets of water entering it at different points provide turbulence, and standing or sitting against them provides a wonderful gentle massage to the body. The combination of heat and water-massage relaxes the muscles and stimulates the whole system so that the bather emerges refreshed and revitalized. It is also great fun since the tub usually accommodates a number of people at once. An outdoor hot tub has the added exhilaration of enabling you to bathe in steaming, fragrant water while you breathe the fresh frosty air of winter or feel snowflakes on your nose!

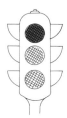 STOP!

STOP! How aware are you of your body's messages *right now*? How are you feeling? Is there tension, stiffness, tiredness in any part of your body? Do you need to get up and stretch? Take some deep breaths? Relax your shoulders? Rest your eyes? Rest your mind? Close your eyes for a minute and take some long, slow deep breaths to enable you to get in touch with your experience. Then respond to what your body is asking you to do.

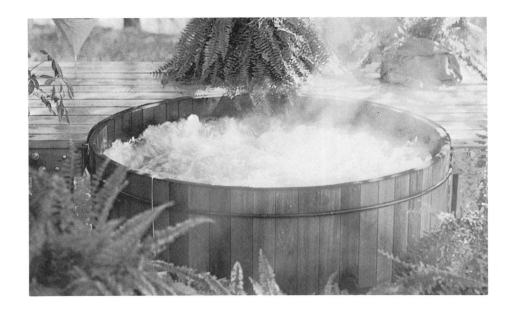

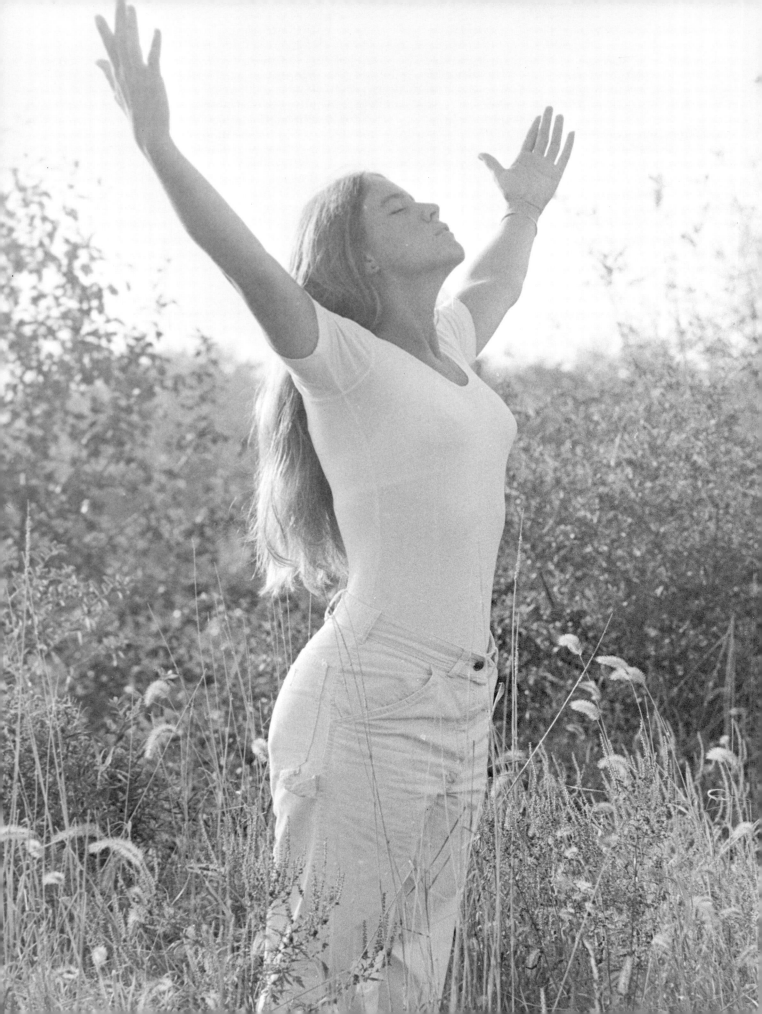

WAY TWO
getting to know and love your body

BEFRIENDING OUR BODIES

"The body is the only vehicle that we have on this earth to experience life and to reach our highest potential."

Where does health begin? In answering that question most of us would undoubtedly say "with the body". Yet, if we look at our lives objectively and honestly, we may see that we don't honor our bodies as much as our belief in their importance would warrant. We expect them to function smoothly and give us no trouble, like a brand new car, and we are surprised and even angry when they break down (sickness). Nevertheless, the signals of the body which can help us to eliminate sickness and disease from our lives are there for us to hear, if we listen. If we can learn to love and care for our bodies in a real way, they will more than repay our care by the quality of life they will allow us to experience.

We need to befriend our bodies; to re-acquaint ourselves with them and respect them; to learn how they function, why they malfunction, what their needs are, and how to provide for those needs. Role models (people who can inspire us with their actions) are significantly lacking in this area of our lives. Most of us have probably known few people in our lives who express the philosophy quoted at the top of this page: that care and respect for the body are essential to our higher growth as individuals. The speaker was Yogi Amrit Desai, founder of the Kripalu Center for Holistic Health.

There are many old sayings in our language which embody this principle: "the body is the temple of the soul", "a healthy mind in a healthy body", etc. Yet we seem somehow to have lost sight of this ancient wisdom and have become overconcerned with intellectual pursuits. This is like trying to build a beautiful house without taking time to lay the foundation properly; the walls are going to sag, the ceilings crack, and eventually the whole structure will come tumbling down!

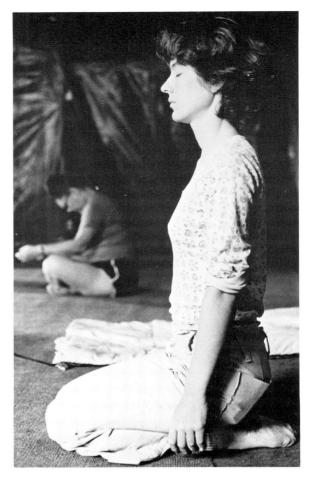

The Kripalu Approach teaches us to begin with the body. This chapter will show you a number of different ways to become re-acquainted with your old and faithful friend, your body, and learn to treat it more lovingly. Whatever your present state of health and mobility, you can improve it quite easily if you know how. This will enrich your whole experience of life. What counts is not how mobile, flexible or agile you are, but rather how sensitive you are to the needs of your body and how caring you are in meeting those needs.

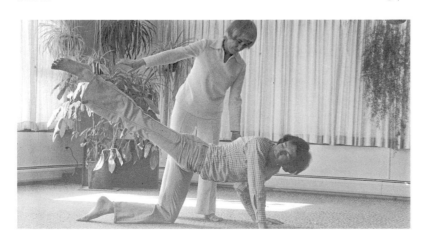

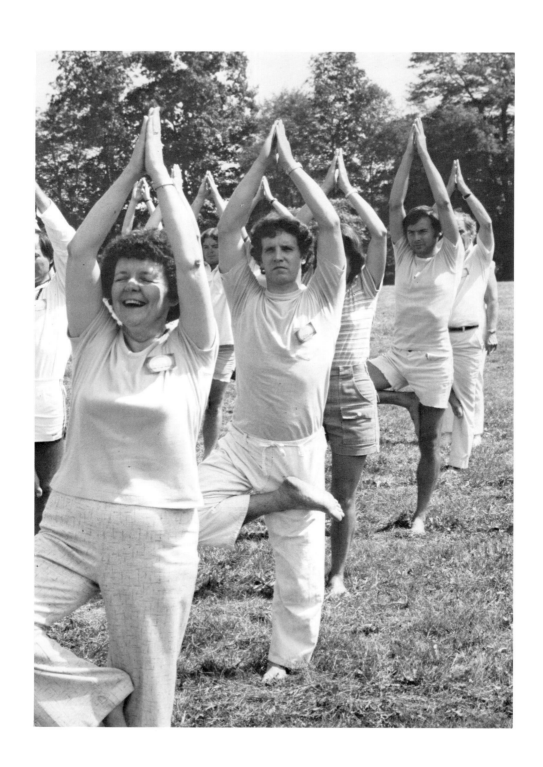

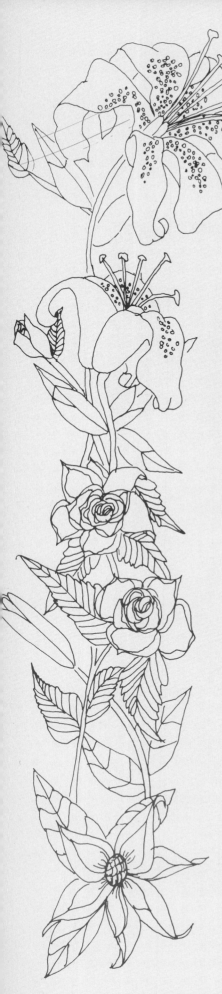

Self–Discovery

How Well Do You Know Your Body?

Awareness

Sit in a comfortable posture, eyes closed, and enter into relaxation by breathing deeply and regularly, and allowing your mind to quiet down. Reflect on each of the following questions, with your eyes closed, after you have read them. Allow the questions to be an experience rather than a thinking process.

1. How does your body feel to you as a rule? Healthy? Fit? Energetic? Sluggish? Supple? Jot down a few words to describe it.

2. Go through your whole body mentally, stopping at each part (head, face, neck, hands, etc.) and trying to feel and visualize it clearly. Notice whether there is any tension or tiredness present, any aches or pains that you were not aware of before you stopped to check it out.

3. Now try to visualize your inner organs (heart, lungs, liver, etc.), your digestive system, your circulatory system, and your breathing mechanism, one after the other. See if you can become more aware of how they are functioning right now. Feel any blockage, any pockets of tension, any irregularity.

Acceptance

Ask yourself:

1. Am I really aware of what is happening in my own body, ongoingly, or do I tend to take it for granted?

2. Am I so busy doing what I'm doing and thinking of other things, that I hardly ever pay attention to how my body is functioning?

3. Does my body have messages for me that I am not able to hear because of the noise in my mind?

Experience 6

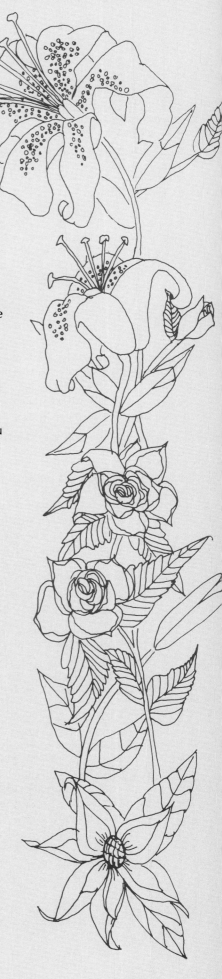

Adjustment

Now that you have become more aware of the miraculous workings of your body that you normally are not attuned to, it makes sense to think of some ways to become more conscious, ongoingly, of what is happening in that body. Ask yourself:

1. What can I do to become more aware of the functioning of my body (e.g. stop from time to time through the day and "check in", take more relaxation, etc.)?

2. What did I notice just now about my body that I need to particularly pay more attention to (e.g. I noticed pain and stiffness in my neck, there seemed to be digestive problems I was not aware of, etc.)?

3. Write down some specific ways in which you can make changes which will help you become more attuned to your body and its needs.

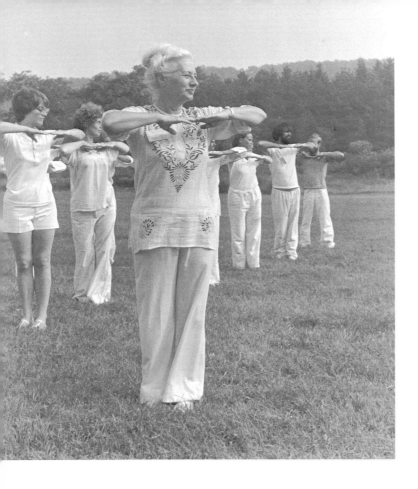

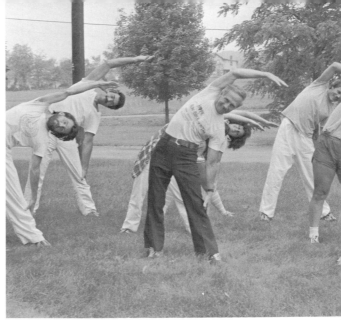

YOGA AND HOLISTIC HEALTH

In the West, yoga is generally known as a system of physical exercise which is used to help slim the body and make it more flexible and youthful, and to calm the mind and free it of tension and worry. But this is merely one branch of yoga known as Hatha Yoga. Yoga is, in fact, a complex science which has many branches. It is one of the most ancient and complete systems of self-development and Holistic Health that the world has known. Both Hatha Yoga postures and the philosophical realizations which go with them emerged spontaneously from the deep meditation experiences of the ancient ascetics of India at least 6,000 years ago. Yoga (which means "union" or "wholeness") was subsequently developed into an extremely precise science, one which is also a great art. Yoga is scientific because it has developed specific, time-tested and proven techniques which have precise and predictable results. It is an art because it needs constant practice for the achievement of perfection and because it is ultimately a highly personal experience and form of self-expression.

Hatha Yoga -- The Gentle Exercise System for All Ages, Shapes and Sizes

Hatha Yoga postures (known as asanas) are very different from other forms of physical exercise. They are designed not so much for muscular development as to bring about the balanced functioning of the nerves and glands. These methods are safe and simple and can be easily grasped and mastered by almost anyone, with consistent practice. As yoga exercises are done in a slow, steady manner, they do not require a great deal of stamina or flexibility. Consequently, they can be practiced and enjoyed by the young and old alike. Those with a physical disease or disability can also benefit from doing yoga; it has even been successfully taught to bedridden older people, and those in wheelchairs! The postures, when done with proper guidance, never produce a strain on the body but rather serve to enhance and stimulate the functioning of the inner organs.

Although Hatha Yoga does work on external physical and emotional problems, its main focus is upon the *root causes* of these problems which are usually found in the functioning of the nerves and glands, or in the mind. Obesity, for example, is not necessarily caused by overeating alone. It can be the result of a malfunctioning thyroid gland, of agitated and tense nerves, or of outdated thinking patterns. Yoga postures work directly on relaxing such deep-set tensions. At the same time, they affect the functioning of the glandular and nervous systems, adding strength, resilience, and harmony. As a result, yoga postures bring about a deep and lasting change in our state of health by focusing on the very source of our physical problems.

The glandular and nervous systems of the body are mainly responsible for controlling our thought patterns, emotional reactions, and our degree of happiness or unhappiness. All physical and mental processes are regulated by the glands and the nerves -- if they are not functioning properly, you may be medically alive, but you are not alive in the true sense of being holistically healthy.

Physical health alone will not satisfy our deeper inner needs. Hatha Yoga is not an end in itself but a means, a stepping stone to higher levels of consciousness. The ultimate purpose of yoga is to unite the forces of "Ha" (positive, masculine energy symbolized by the sun) and "Tha" (negative, feminine energy symbolized by the moon). These complementary energies exist within each of us and give rise to our experience of polarity, of conflict, as we live in the world. When the energies of "Ha" and "Tha" are united within us through the practice of yoga, it is possible for us to transcend these apparent conflicts and to experience the essential unity of all life. When practiced in its true sense, yoga dissolves the polarity in which we usually live and becomes a tool for us to enter a higher state of consciousness where we live in harmony with all that surrounds us.

TYPES OF YOGA

Most people begin their yoga practice with Hatha Yoga, but there are other forms of yoga that lead towards this goal of integration of body, mind and spirit. These other forms of yoga practice are described in the first written compilations of yogic knowledge, Patanjali's *Yoga Sutras,* composed about 200 B.C., and are outlined below:

Karma Yoga - wholeness through service, work and action

Jnana Yoga - wholeness through knowledge and study.

Bhakti Yoga - wholeness through devotion and selfless love.

Mantra Yoga - wholeness through sound vibration and speech.

Raja Yoga - wholeness through control of the mind.

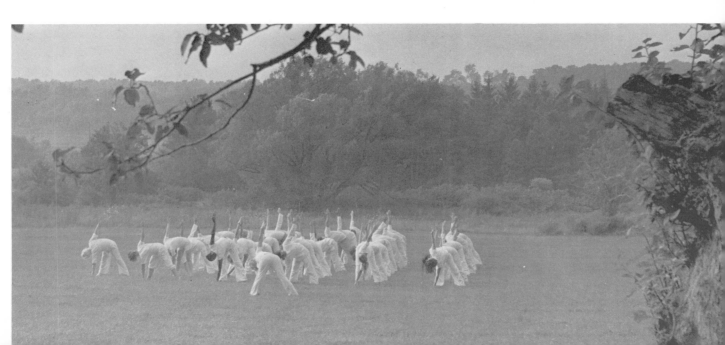

TEN EASY YOGA POSTURES

Like any other form of exercise, yoga postures are best practiced after some limbering-up has taken place to warm up the body and loosen the muscles. The first series of movements suggested here are for that purpose. Called the "Wake-up Routine" because it is a wonderful way to wake up in the early morning, these simple movements are also an excellent way to start your yoga practice.

As with all yoga postures, carry the movements out slowly and gently, without any strain. You should make a moderate effort to stretch your body a little more than usual, but never to the point of extreme discomfort or pain. The purpose is to experience your body and its capabilities, and to enjoy the pleasant feeling of stretching, like a cat or a small child. Remember that you are not competing with anyone, not even yourself. You do not need to perform the postures "perfectly" but rather to feel your body in new ways, with a new awareness, and learn from what it is telling you. As much as possible, do these postures with your eyes closed, as this will heighten your sense of contact with your body and your level of relaxation.

NOTE:
The postures have been presented in a specific order so that each bend in one direction is followed by a complementary bend in the opposite direction. It is advisable to always do two complementary postures, as it balances the body.

Limbering Up

Waking up in the morning is like the birth of a baby -- it can thrust you into the world abruptly, even jarringly, or it can be a gentle loving entry into the daylight which will keep you calm, serene and centered all day long.

The key is to move slowly, allowing your body time to make the delicate transition from the sleeping, passive mode to the alert, active state. Muscles and joints that have stiffened during the night's inactivity must be gently stretched and mobilized, particularly the spine. The body energy needs to be stimulated gently. The lungs need to be opened up so that you again inhale deeply and fully after a night of shallow breathing, when the body required less oxygen.

The Waking-Up Routine

INSTRUCTIONS

1. Remain in bed (if your bed is not too soft) or gently rise and lie on the floor beside the bed. Lie on your back with legs straight and arms comfortably at your sides. Relax.

2. Clasp your hands on your stomach, interlacing the fingers. Invert your palms stretching them downwards, toward your feet, and straightening your arms. Now slowly (all these movements should be very slow unless otherwise indicated) begin to lift your arms into the air, breathing in deeply and slowly, and bring them down to the floor or bed behind/above your head, fully stretched out. Exhaling, stretch and arch your back, loosening up your spine.

3. Unclasp your hands, exhaling, and as you inhale, stretch the right arm and the right leg in a straight line, making that side of your body longer than the other and lifting your right hip slightly. Relax, exhaling. Now repeat with your left arm and leg. Stretch fully and inhale deeply, lifting your left hip.

4. Lift your arms again until your hands are directly above your shoulders (toward the ceiling). Release your hands and gently rotate them around the wrists, several times in each direction, making complete circles.

5. Gently lower your arms to the sides until they rest on the floor and are directly out from your shoulders. Inhaling, slowly raise your right knee, sliding the right foot along the ground until it is next to your left knee. Exhaling, slowly twist your body, bringing your right knee over towards the ground on the outside of your left thigh and turning your head to the right. *Don't strain.* Be very relaxed and enjoy the stretch. Breathe deeply in the position. Now, exhaling slowly, return to center, and slide your foot back to its starting position beside the other foot. Relax for a moment, breathing deeply. Now, inhaling, repeat the twist on the other side. Relax.

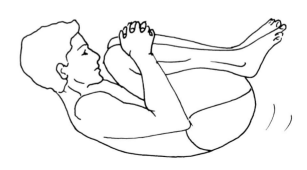

6. For this step you will need to be on the floor, with a little space around you. Gently come to a seated position, with your knees up to your chest, feet on the floor, hands clasped under your knees, back rounded and head bent forward. Begin to gently roll back onto your upper back, *keeping the spine well curved, and the head tucked in* (this is important). Rock back and forth like this about a dozen times, fairly briskly so that the momentum going back will help you come forward. Straighten your legs as you rock back; bend them again as you return. Breathe in as you rock back, out as you rock forward. Then relax on your back.

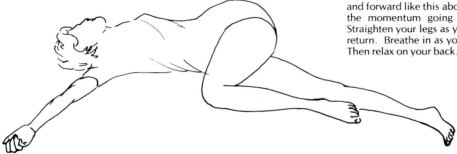

1. The Triangle (Trikonasana)

BENEFITS:

1. Provides alternate flexing and relaxing of the trunk's lateral and dorsal muscles, promoting resilience in the spine and proper placement in the bones and muscles of the hips.

2. Invigorates the abdominal muscles and organs.

3. Tones the hamstring muscles and strengthens the sciatic nerves.

INSTRUCTIONS:

Triangle 1:

1. Stand with your legs about shoulder width apart, feet turned slightly outward. Exhale.

2. Inhale as you raise both arms sideways until they are in line with your shoulders, with palms facing down.

3. Exhale as you bend to your left, from your waist, pushing your right hip slightly to the right. Stretch your right arm parallel to the floor, over your head, keeping it close to your ear. Allow your left hand to glide along your thigh, toward your ankle, as far as comfortable. Keep the legs straight and pelvis forward. Do not twist at the waist, shoulders, or legs.

4. Inhaling, slowly raise up to the original position.

5. Repeat to the opposite side, bending sideways to the right.

6. Raise up to the standing position.

7. Exhale as you lower your arms and bring your feet together. Relax.

Triangle 2:

1. Stand as in Triangle I. Exhale.

2. As you inhale, raise your arms sideways to shoulder level with your palms facing down.

3. As you exhale, twist your upper body to the left, then bend and lower your right hand to the outside of your left foot. Your left arm remains stretched in line with your right arm. Turn your head and look at your left thumb. Keep your legs straight. Hold to comfort level.

4. Inhale as you return to standing and bring your arms in line with your shoulders.

5. Exhale as you turn your upper body to face the front.

6. Repeat in the opposite direction.

7. As you exhale, lower your arms and bring your feet together. Relax.

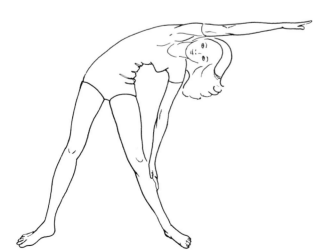

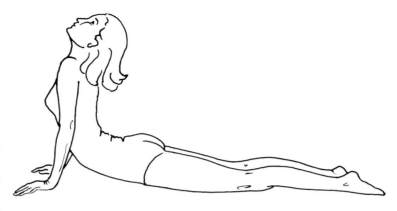

2. The Cobra (Bhujangasana)

BENEFITS:

1. Helps to regulate the functions of the gonads and uterus, and to prevent and relieve menstrual disorders.

2. Stimulates and relaxes vertebrae from the neck to the base of the spine. Strengthens and tones weak spinal muscles.

3. Recharges the entire abdominal region with an abundant flow of blood. Rejuvenates the kidneys. Stimulates the thyroid and adrenal glands. Trims abdominal fat and tones the buttocks.

4. Helps to relieve the tension of backache caused by long hours of sitting, walking or driving. An excellent posture to do before going to sleep at night.

HINTS & PRECAUTIONS:

As with all yoga postures, sudden or jerking movements may cause stiffness. Train your body gently through consistent practice rather than by forcing or fighting it. You should rise up to the Cobra position using only the muscles of your back and not your arms. You may want to place your palms on the back of your thighs and rise up with no support. The Cobra should not be done after the third month of pregnancy.

INSTRUCTIONS:

1. Lie on your abdomen and relax completely. Place your forehead on the floor, palms down, fingertips in line with your shoulders. Keep your elbows off the floor and your legs together with the toes pointed. Exhale deeply.

2. Inhaling, slowly and gracefully raise your forehead, nose and chin, followed by your shoulders and chest, in one continuous movement. Use your arms to maintain your balance, but not for support. Keep your elbows bent and your shoulders down, not hunched.

3. Arch your head back and look up. Your navel and hips must remain on the floor. Hold the position, remaining relaxed.

4. Exhaling, slowly uncurl your spine and lower your chest, chin, nose and then eyes until your forehead rests again on the floor.

5. Repeat the Cobra 2 or 3 times.

3. The Head-To-Knee Posture (Paschimottanasana)

BENEFITS:

1. Stretches and strengthens the nerves of the lower back, thereby helping to prevent functional disorders of the stomach, liver, spleen, kidneys and intestines.

2. Improves lost appetite and stimulates an underactive liver and kidneys. Helps to relieve constipation and indigestion.

3. Streamlines the abdomen. Slims and tones hips and thighs.

4. Helps prevent hemorrhoids.

5. Provides a powerful stretch for the entire back, from the neck to the heels.

6. Develops and tones the back and the hamstring muscles of the legs.

7. Promotes elasticity of the spine and strengthens the vital nerve plexuses of the spine. Stretches and strengthens the crucial sciatic nerve.

HINTS & CAUTIONS:

Avoid sudden movements and strain, as in every yoga posture. Do not force your head to touch your knees if this is very uncomfortable or painful. Simply come as close as you can without strain and you will still gain all the benefits. Concentrate on bending from the lower back rather than from the shoulders and upper back. Your knees should be straight in order to derive full benefit from this posture. If you suffer from any back injury or from severe constipation, practice this posture cautiously, increasing the holding time very gradually.

INSTRUCTIONS:

1. Sit with both legs stretched out in front of you, on the floor, and your back straight. Exhale deeply.

2. Inhaling, slowly raise your arms above your head without bending your elbows. Stretch upwards from the waist.

3. Exhaling, bend from the hips, stretching forward over your knees. Bring your head as close as you comfortably can to your knees. Hold onto your feet, ankles, calves, or wherever you can reach comfortably without straining. Breathe deeply.

4. Inhaling, slowly sit up again, stretching your arms above your head.

5. Exhaling, lower your arms gracefully. Relax, breathing deeply.

An easier, beginner's version is to bend one leg, placing the sole of your foot against the inside of the opposite leg, as high on the leg as possible. Then bend forward over your outstretched leg, following the same steps already listed for the Head-to-Knee posture. Be sure that the straightened leg remains flat on the floor and straight forward from the hip (not slanted out). Repeat on the other side.

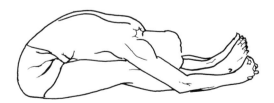

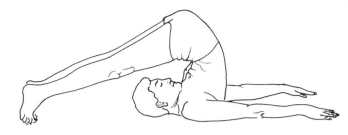

4. The Plough (Halasana)

BENEFITS:

1. Aligns the vertebrae and brings a fresh supply of blood to the nerve centers along the spine. An ideal orthopedic exercise, helping to correct spinal irregularities in children and minor dislocations of the vertebrae in adults.

2. Enhances body symmetry and strengthens the back muscles.

3. Rejuvenates and cleanses the gonads (sex glands) and pancreas, liver, spleen, kidneys and adrenal glands.

4. Helps regulate the function of the thyroid, calming the nerves and blessing the entire system with youthfulness.

5. Helps relieve exhaustion, fatigue and stiffness of the back and shoulders.

6. Diminishes facial lines and wrinkles.

7. Aids in the treatment of diabetes and menstrual disorders.

8. Trims away accumulated fat in the abdomen and hips. Tones and firms the legs.

9. Strengthens the organs of the neck and thorax.

10. Stimulates brain activity, relieving headaches and disorders caused by anemia of the brain. Increases blood circulation to the brain and clears the mind.

HINTS AND CAUTIONS:

Again, be careful not to strain by overly-vigorous movements. Do not attempt to force your toes to the floor; it is not necessary. If the Plough is difficult for you, try this preparation: lie on the floor with the top of your head about 1½ feet from a wall. As your feet come over your head into the Plough, brace them against the wall then simply walk down the wall to the floor. You can also rock into the Plough position.

INSTRUCTIONS:

1. Lying on your back, place your arms close to your sides, palms down. Keep both knees straight. Exhale.

2. Inhaling, press your palms against the floor and slowly raise your legs until they point to the ceiling.

3. Exhaling, lower your legs over your head until your feet touch the floor behind your head, or come as close as is comfortable. Do not bend your knees.

4. Hold this position, supporting your hips with your hands if necessary to maintain balance. Breathe deeply and slowly.

5. Inhaling, slowly lower your back, vertebra by vertebra, until your hips have reached the floor and your legs are toward the ceiling once more. Exhaling, slowly lower your legs to the floor without bending your knees. (Beginners: bend your knees towards your forehead and press your hands into the ground until your upper back is on the floor. Then straighten the legs again and lower them slowly.)

Relax and breathe normally, experiencing the benefits.

5. The Shoulderstand (Sarvangasana)

BENEFITS:

1. Helps to regulate both over and underweight by normalizing the functions of the thyroid and parathyroid glands, through the pressure of the chin. These glands regulate metabolic processes, heartbeat and blood pressure. Every vital organ is affected by the well-being of the thyroid gland.

2. Sends a generous supply of blood to the organs in the upper portion of the body, helping to prevent and relieve such ailments as throat and chest colds, sore throats, bronchitis, asthma and headaches. The heart is relieved of the strain of pumping blood against gravity to the demanding organs of the head and neck.

3. Improves circulation, relieving pressure on the blood vessels and making them resilient. Helps prevent and relieve varicose veins and hemorrhoids.

4. Helps to correct displacement of vital internal glands and organs, especially the female organs. Benefits those suffering from female disorders.

5. Tones the gonads (sex glands), helping to maintain the vitality of the entire body. Helps restore dissipated energy, bringing new youth to the entire system.

6. Effectively combats insomnia, nervous disorders and hypertension, as well as sluggishness and indolence, by regulating glandular functions.

7. Eases constipation and indigestion.

8. Nourishes facial skin, scalp, and hair roots, helping to erase wrinkles, and improving general complexion.

9. Regulates the thymus gland, which is the source of physical and mental development. Highly recommended for growing children and adolescents.

10. Note the Reverse Posture, given as a preparation for the Shoulderstand, primarily benefits the gonads and sends increased circulation to the face.

HINTS AND CAUTIONS:

The Shoulderstand is a most precious gift, given to humanity by the ancient yogis. Its Sanskrit name means "the exercise that benefits the entire body". It produces many of the rejuvenating effects of the more difficult inverted postures. Persons suffering from extremely high or low blood pressure, organic thyroid disorders, chronic nasal catarrh, glaucoma, detached retina or weak eye capillaries, should consult their physician before attempting the Shoulderstand.

INSTRUCTIONS:

First, an easy version: The Reverse Posture

1. Lie on your back with your hands at your sides, palms facing down, your feet together and legs straight. Exhale deeply.

2. Inhaling, slowly raise your straightened legs toward the ceiling.

3. Exhaling, lift your hips and lower your legs toward the floor over your head. Inhaling, lift your legs at a sixty degree angle. Support your hips with your hands. Hold the position. Breathe deeply.

4. Exhaling, lower your legs toward the floor over your head. Then, inhaling, slowly and steadily lower your back to the floor. Exhaling again, return your legs to the floor. Relax. (Beginners: Bend your knees toward your forehead and press your hands into the ground. When your upper back is on the floor, stretch your legs and gently lower them slowly toward the floor.)

The Shoulderstand (after 1 week of practice of the Reverse Posture)

1. Lie on your back, as for the Reverse Posture. Press down on the floor with your palms. Inhaling, gradually raise your straightened legs to a perpendicular position, keeping your knees straight.

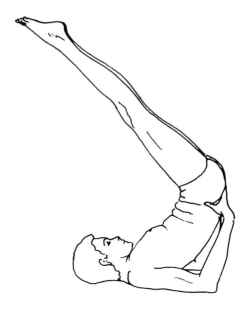

2. Exhaling, slowly raise your hips and lower your legs over your head. Support your upper back with your hands, bringing your entire body into a vertical position as you inhale. Point your toes toward the ceiling. Make your body as straight as possible.

3. While holding this position, keep your chin firmly pressed against your breastbone. Breathe deeply.

4. Exhaling, lower your legs over your head. Inhaling, lower your back to the floor, reversing your upward movement. Finally, exhaling, bring your legs back to the floor. Do not repeat immediately. Relax and breathe deeply.

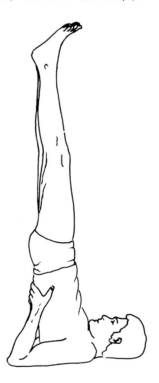

6. The Fish (Matsyasana)

BENEFITS:

1. Helps to correct lung displacement in the thoracic cavity caused by restricted and long immobilization (such as sitting at desks) thus increasing lung capacity. Helps prevent and relieve asthma.

2. Eases curved and stiffened backs.

3. Flushes muscles of the spine, as well as the abdominal and neck organs. Excellent for colds and swollen tonsils.

4. Increases circulation to the back and stimulates the nerves of the spinal cord, sympathetic nervous sytem and the solar plexus.

5. Tones the abdominal viscera (the liver, spleen and pelvic organs).

6. Helps alleviate painful hemorrhoids.

7. Benefits the adrenal glands, gonads and pancreas.

8. Tones the chest and back, improving posture and thus affecting psychological attitude.

HINTS & CAUTIONS:

The Fish is often done immediately following the Shoulderstand, as it both complements and stabilizes the stretch given to the neck muscles by the Shoulderstand.

INSTRUCTIONS:

1. Lie on your back with your legs tucked underneath your buttocks, and your arms resting at your sides. Relax, and exhale deeply.

2. Inhaling, using your elbows for support, arch your back between your hips and the top of your head. Rest the top of your head on the floor (beginners may find it easier to place the hands palms down under the hips and arch up with the support of the elbows).

3. Hold the posture. Breathe deeply. If you feel secure, lift your elbows and join your hands over your chest in the prayer position.

4. Exhaling, bring your arms out of the prayer position and place your elbows on the floor for support. Then gently lower your head and then your back, supporting your body with your elbows. Release your hands and relax. Do not repeat the Fish a second time.

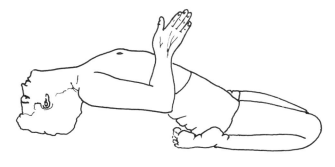

7. The Twist (Ardha Matsyendrasana)

BENEFITS:

1. Helps prevent lumbago, backstrain, and certain forms of sciatica.

2. Tones sluggish kidneys and adrenals, aiding in the process of diuresis.

3. Decongests a clogged liver and spleen. Combats obesity, constipation and indigestion by increasing the peristaltic movement of the bowels.

4. Helps relieve asthma.

5. Removes calcium deposits of the shoulders, freeing shoulder movement. Helps overcome stiffness of the neck.

6. Strengthens and elasticizes the spine: helps correct stooped shoulders, bent back, defective posture and minor spinal deformities.

INSTRUCTIONS:

First Easy Version: The Half Twist

1. Sit with your legs stretched before you. Bend your right leg, placing the sole of your right foot on the floor to the left of your left knee.

2. Place your left palm on the floor behind your back on the left side Point your fingers away from your body. Keep your back very straight and your arm as close as possible to your back.

3. Place your right arm along the inside of your right leg. Grasp your right ankle. Exhale deeply.

4. Sitting erect and inhaling, turn slowly to the left until you are looking at the back wall. Hold the position, breathing deeply. Do not change the upright position of your right knee.

5. Exhaling, release the posture slowly. Relax.

6. Repeat in the opposite direction.

7. Repeat for a total of two or three times in each direction.

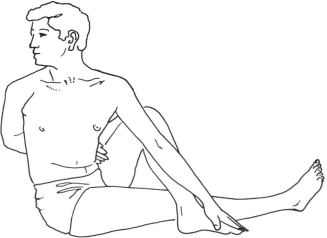

Version Two: The Full Twist (after 3-4 weeks of practice of the Half Twist).

1. Sit on your heels.

2. Shift your hips so that you are sitting on the floor, to the left of both feet.

3. Grasp your right ankle with the right hand and place it on the outside of your left knee. Keep the back straight and the knee upright.

4. Raise your arms so that they are perpendicular to your body.

5. Now, inhaling, twist to the right. Bring your left arm to the right (outside) of your right knee and clasp the right ankle or foot with your left hand. Place the right hand on the floor behind and very close to your back, with your fingers pointing away from your body.

6. Now look over your right shoulder, twisting from the base of your spine up to your neck. Hold this position. Placing gentle pressure on your right (raised) leg with your left elbow will increase the twist.

7. Exhaling, slowly return to your starting position. Release the position and relax.

8. Repeat in opposite direction.

8. Yoga Mudra

BENEFITS:

1. Expands the lungs and stimulates the lung cells.

2. Stimulates the peristaltic movement of the bowels, helping to relieve constipation.

3. Strengthens the nerves and muscles of the abdominal and pelvic areas.

4. Recharges the colon and intestinal nerves, aligning the abdominal organs by an external and internal massage.

5. Develops the chest and bust, and exercises seldom-used arm and shoulder muscles.

6. Provides relief for tension throughout the trunk area caused by extended periods of sitting and bending.

7. Improves general posture, thus increasing self-confidence.

HINTS AND CAUTIONS:

If you suffer from chronic constipation, practice this posture gently, releasing it slowly and avoiding jerky movements.

INSTRUCTIONS:

1. Assume a kneeling position, placing your palms on your knees. Exhale deeply.

2. Inhaling, bring your arms behind your back in a slow and steady circular motion. Interlock your fingers and straighten your arms. Do not change the position of your palms.

3. Exhaling, bend forward, raising your arms as high as possible, until your forehead touches the floor.

4. Hold the position. For an additional stretch you may bring your chin to the floor.

5. Inhaling, sit up slowly. Exhaling, let your arms return to your knees on their own accord. (The spontaneous movement you may experience at this stage is a preliminary experience of prana-directed movement.)

6. Repeat the posture a second time.

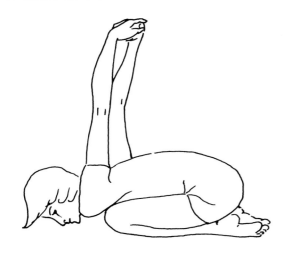

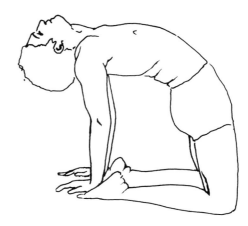

9. The Camel (Ushtrasana)

BENEFITS:

1. Eases back tension and increases spinal flexibility. Helps to correct a curved back and rounded shoulders.

2. Develops the chest and bust, firming the muscles of the upper arms, thighs and abdomen.

3. Strengthens and elasticizes the feet.

4. Gently massages the heart.

5. Rejuvenates the thyroid and gonads, bestowing youthfulness on your entire system.

HINTS AND CAUTIONS:

As back stretching is difficult for many people, proceed slowly. Avoid tensing your muscles as this will inhibit both flexibility and gradual, graceful movement. If you are suffering from a hernia, do not practice the Camel.

INSTRUCTIONS:

1. Assume a kneeling position. Place your palms on your knees. Exhale deeply.

2. Inhaling, slowly bring your arms behind your back. Place your palms on the floor, directly behind your feet. Point your fingers away from your body.

3. Exhaling, shift your weight to your arms, dropping your head back.

4. Inhaling, raise your hips and arch your back. Shift your body weight *onto* your knees and thighs.

5. Hold the posture to comfort level. Breathe deeply.

6. Exhaling, lower your hips to your heels. Keep your hands on the floor and your head back.

7. Inhaling, raise your head and shoulders.

8. Exhaling, slowly bring your hands onto your knees. Relax. Repeat 2 to 3 times.

10. The Sun Salutation (Surya Namaskar)

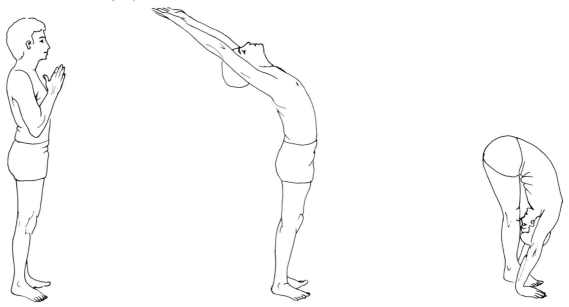

INSTRUCTIONS:

1. Stand erect with your feet and legs together. Join your palms in the prayer position in front of your chest, with your elbows pointed downward. Interlock your thumbs.

2. Without releasing your hands, slowly raise your arms over your head as you inhale. Keeping your head between your arms, bend slightly backward with breath held. Keep your knees locked and your feet firmly positioned on the floor.

3. Exhaling, bend forward from the hips, placing your hands palms down on the floor on either side of your feet, with your toes and fingertips in a straight line. If this is too difficult, you may bend your knees slightly.

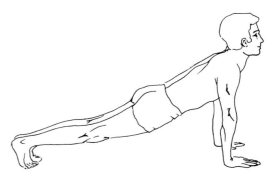

5. Hold your breath as you straighten your right knee and bring your left leg back to join it. Both feet and legs should be together. Straighten your arms with your palms still on the floor so that your entire body forms a straight line (the push-up position).

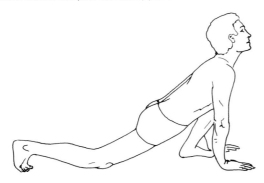

4. Inhaling, stretch your right leg behind you as far as possible. Rest your right knee on the floor and curl your toes under your foot. Your left foot should remain stationary between your hands, with your chest touching your left thigh and knee. Look up and arch your back, stretching your head, neck and chest.

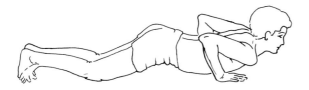

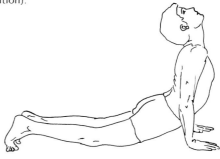

6. Exhaling, gradually lower your body touching your knees, chest, and forehead to the floor. If it is difficult to place the forehead on the floor, you can touch the chin instead. The buttocks remain raised.

7. Inhale and lower your hips and abdomen to the floor, uncurling your toes and relaxing your head, neck and chest. Arching your back as in the Cobra, straighten your arms and rest your weight on your hands. The hips and thighs should remain on the floor.

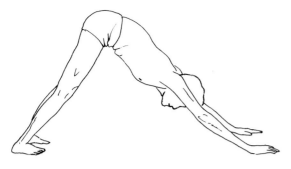

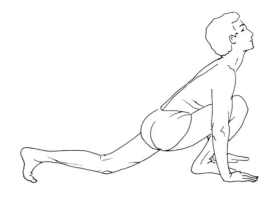

8. Curl your toes under your feet once again. Exhaling, lift your hips, resting your weight on your hands and feet. Your body should form a triangle, with your head between your arms. Keep your feet flat on the floor by pressing your heels down. If this is difficult, walk toward the hands until your feet are flat. Press your torso toward your legs, so that your spine curves inward.

9. Inhaling, take a long and quick step forward, and place your right foot between your hands. Keep your left leg stretched behind you and lower your left knee to the floor. Then raise your head and arch your back (this position reverses step #4).

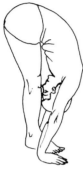

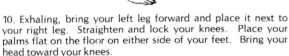

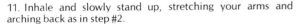

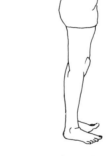

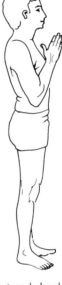

10. Exhaling, bring your left leg forward and place it next to your right leg. Straighten and lock your knees. Place your palms flat on the floor on either side of your feet. Bring your head toward your knees.

11. Inhale and slowly stand up, stretching your arms and arching back as in step #2.

12. Exhaling, gradually lower your arms back to the prayer position. Stand still with your eyes closed for a few seconds.

BENEFITS:

1. Tones the digestive system by alternately stretching and compressing the abdominal region. Massages the liver, stomach, spleen, intestines and kidneys. Stimulates the digestive process and helps to relieve constipation and dyspepsia.

2. Thoroughly ventilates the lungs. Oxygenates the blood and removes carbon dioxide and other toxic gases from the respiratory tract.

3. Increases circulation throughout the entire system. Brings warmth, vigor and vitality to the limbs of the body.

4. Stretches and massages the spinal column, toning and regulating functions of the sympathetic and parasympathetic nervous systems. Helps dispel insomnia, hypertension, worry and anxiety. Improves the memory.

5. Helps normalize the functions of the endocrine glands, thereby relieving emotional stress and tension. The thyroid gland is especially benefited by the Sun Salutation.

6. Refreshes and tones the skin, helping to remove premature wrinkles and prevent sagging.

7. Strengthens and tones all the muscles of the body, especially those in the back. Helps relieve and prevent backaches caused by long hours of standing or sitting.

8. Tones and firms the upper arms, bust and shoulders. Effectively helps to correct posture and bestow a sense of balance, grace and self-confidence.

9. Affects activity in the uterus and ovaries, helping to regulate the menstrual cycle. Relieves and prevents menstrual discomfort. Facilitates easy childbirth.

10. Tones and slims the waist, thighs, hips and buttocks. Helps remove excess weight from any area of the body which may be improperly proportioned as a result of overeating or lack of exercise.

11. Helps to prevent the loss of hair and slows the greying process.

12. Affects each cell of the body, bestowing an overall feeling of well-being, vitality, and peace. As a result, the mind is able to function with greater clarity and calmness.

HINTS AND CAUTIONS:

This exercise is traditionally practiced in the early morning as a salute to the sun, nature's symbol of health and long life. It is a combination of asanas and breathing exercises which, when mastered, produces a meditative flow of bodily movement. The Sun Salutation may be used as a warm-up before your daily yoga exercises, as it limbers the spine as well as all of the muscles of the body and invigorates the entire system.

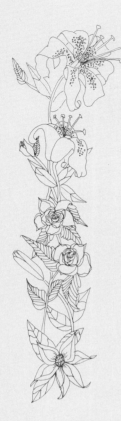

Self-Discovery Experience 7

Are You Really Breathing?

Close your eyes when you've read this paragraph, and *observe* your breathing (it is not necessary to change it, just observe). Is it shallow or deep? Slow or fast? Regular or irregular? How are you sitting? And how does that affect your breathing? How do you feel -- sleepy and lazy, alert and vigorous? Is the air around you warm or cool? Fresh or stuffy? Dry or moist? Become very clearly aware of these answers before you read on.

YOGIC BREATHING AND PRANA

Life and Breath

Breathing is the most basic function of human life, for what we call life begins with our first breath in and ends with our last breath out. Life is the process contained between these two breaths and sustained by the intervening breaths. Breath, then, is life, for although we can survive for many days without food and water, without breathing we can survive for only a few minutes.

Because the relationship between breath and life itself is so intimate, our way of breathing has a profound effect on the quality of our lives. Yet how many of us are aware of our manner of breathing at any given moment? Or of how it is affecting our body, mind and emotions? The act of breathing, for most of us, is an automatic process which we take completely for granted until a problem develops.

"Normal" breathing is usually a shallow, superficial process involving just the upper portion of the lungs, and using only a small percentage of their 5-quart capacity. This poor breathing habit has developed from several causes. In childhood, many of us learned that good posture meant tucking in our stomachs and pushing out our chests (try it and see how it constricts the muscles that allow you to breathe). A second cause is the mostly sedentary lives many of us lead. Third, we all suffer, to some extent, from accumulated tensions and worries which cause the abdomen to become tight, preventing us from inhaling deeply. This shallow, superficial breathing deprives the body of both oxygen and prana (which is mainly supplied to the body through the vehicle of oxygen), bringing about gradual deterioration in health and premature aging.

Pranayama -- the Science of Breath

Pranayama is the yogic science of gaining mastery over prana through special breathing techniques and through making breathing a more conscious process. Since all the functions of the body, voluntary and involuntary, are governed by prana, this "control of prana" means improved functioning of all our organs and systems: respiratory, circulatory, digestive, glandular and nervous. This results in greater resistance to disease, greater calmness and more productivity.

Our mental processes, too, depend on the amount of prana we take in. The regular practice of pranayama dramatically increases mental clarity and concentration. Creative, intellectual and intuitive capacities are also greatly improved. Pranayama is generally taught in yoga classes along with yoga postures. It forms an even more integral part of the Kripalu Approach to yoga, as the following section will demonstrate.

Pranayama also facilitates meditation, because it establishes health and harmony of body and mind, allowing us to transcend both and enter into deeper states of consciousness.

Pranayama has a profound effect upon our emotions, as well as on our physical and mental states, because breathing corresponds closely to emotion. (Notice how you breathe when you are very angry or fearful, as compared to when you are relaxed and about to fall asleep.) Pranayama teaches us how to use our breathing to transform negative or self-destructive emotions into positive growth. Once we can maintain a relaxed breathing pattern when we are angry or tense, we are breaking a chain reaction. If our breath pattern does not transmit a message of tension to our nervous system, the emotion will fail to leave its energy-draining stamp of stress on the body and mind. Usually, our emotions go unnoticed until they have become so overpowering that they are difficult to control.

Pranayama can also be extremely helpful in reducing smoking or overeating. People who smoke often report feeling tense and restless. This tension begins with the pattern of shallow breathing. Yet the need to smoke comes, in part, from the need to take in fuller, deeper breaths to relieve tension. The act of smoking, however, does not fulfill the need for deeper breathing.

It only increases the negative cycle of shallow breathing which creates more tension, followed by more need to smoke.

Pranayama helps with overeating in much the same way. Overeating is a need of the mind and emotions, not of the stomach. Overeating temporarily relieves tension and unpleasant feelings such as loneliness, inadequacy and insecurity. Yogic breathing helps to reduce the need to overeat by balancing the metabolism and calming the mind. The regular practice of pranayama will lead you into a state of relaxation and vigorous, holistic health by helping to balance and harmonize body, mind and emotions. In this way, you are gaining the keys to life itself.

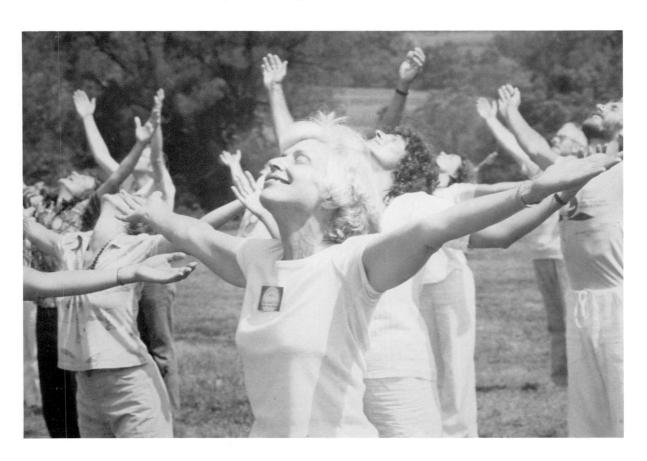

HOW TO DO YOGIC BREATHING

Step 1. Abdominal Breathing

Stand, sit or preferably lie, in a very relaxed position. Breathe in slowly through your nose as you expand your abdomen. Imagine that you have a balloon inside and as you inhale you are slowly inflating it, causing the abdominal area to slowly swell. Feel your diaphragm being pushed down and relaxing.

Breathe out slowly through your nose as you pull your abdominal muscles in, without straining, so that you press all of the air out of your lungs. Continue breathing in as the abdomen rises and out as it falls, until you've established a natural rhythm.

HINT: Place your hands on your abdomen, just above the navel, with fingertips pointing towards each other and just touching. If you are breathing correctly, as you inhale your hands will rise with your abdomen and your finger tips will separate. As you exhale, they will touch again.

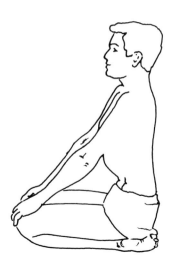

Step 2. "Sounding" Breath

After you are comfortable with abdominal breathing, you are ready to add the next step. In the back of the throat (where there is a small flap of flesh at the back of the soft palate) is the muscle that you use to gargle or snore. Imitate gargling and find the point where the sound originates.

Use that muscle to draw the air into your lungs as you inhale and to control its outward flow as you exhale. Continue abdominal breathing, through your nose (never breathe through the mouth).

You will hear the air being drawn through the throat much like the sound you hear when you press a large seashell to your ear. This sound is not made by the voice, but by contraction of the throat. It is the sound you make through the mouth when you are fogging a mirror. You can learn to make this same sound while breathing in and out through the nose. Abdominal breathing is much easier when you inhale and exhale in this manner because you can control and extend the air flow.

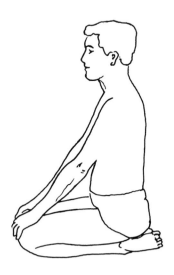

Step 3. Full Yogic Breathing

When you are comfortable doing the abdominal breathing with the sound, you are ready to add the last step: Full Yogic Breathing.

Follow the same steps listed for abdominal breathing. However, now imagine that your lungs are divided into two parts: the upper half (upper chest) and the lower half (the part you are already using in abdominal breathing).

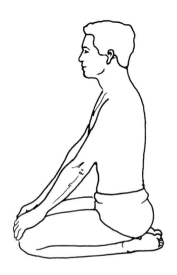

As you inhale, fill the bottom half of the lungs (abdominal breathing) first and then continue to inhale, filling the top half. As you exhale, empty the top half of the lungs first and then empty the bottom half.

Imagine yourself filling a hot water bottle with water. The water enters and fills the bottom first and finally reaches the top. Then as you empty it, the water flows out first from the top and gradually down to the last drops remaining in the bottom, and the sides of the bottle contract together.

Posture is an important part of correct breathing. For your lungs to be free from compression and able to fill fully, your back should be straight but relaxed, with shoulders down, back and loose; your chin should be parallel to the ground and slightly tucked. Make sure your knees are unlocked and not tense.

Benefits: Practice this Full Yogic Breathing as often as you can. It will provide more oxygenation of the blood, resulting in greater relaxation, better emotional balance and control, greater mental clarity and acuity, and greatly improved general health. Your lung capacity will gradually increase, so that you will be less easily winded by exertion. Even chronic lung and bronchial problems will be aided.

HOW TO DO ALTERNATE NOSTRIL BREATHING (Anuloma Viloma)

Alternate Nostril Breathing is the most powerful and beneficial of the various pranayamas (yogic breathing techniques). Its primary purpose is to soothe, purify and strengthen the nervous system. Other benefits include developing control of the body, mind and emotions; increasing mental alertness; cleansing and opening the nasal passages; normalizing the metabolic processes; and helping to combat the overall detrimental effects of daily stress. Alternate Nostril Breathing also helps to establish a balanced breath pattern, believed by the ancient yogis to be important in maintaining overall health.

To do Alternate Nostril Breathing, you should be fairly comfortable with yogic deep breathing (already described).

1. Assume a comfortable sitting position (in a chair or cross-legged on the floor) with your back straight. Sitting on a firm pillow or cushion may help you to hold the position comfortably.

2. Using the right hand, press the index and middle fingers against the palm of the hand, holding out the thumb and last two fingers. The thumb will be used to close one nostril and the last two fingers to close the other nostril. With practice this hand position will become quite comfortable.

3. Using regular, slow Yogic Deep Breathing, close the right nostril and inhale through the left until the lungs are comfortably full. Then close off both nostrils and hold your breath. When you need to exhale, open the right nostril and exhale through that side alone. As soon as the lungs are completely empty, inhale again through the right, hold, then exhale again through the left. This comprises one round of Alternate Nostril Breathing (in left, hold, out right, in right, hold, out left). Practice it until you become accustomed to the pattern.

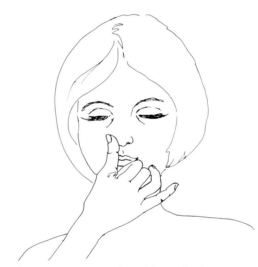

4. When you are comfortable with the pattern of Alternate Nostril Breathing, begin to count mentally, to time each inhalation, hold, and exhalation. At first attempt to get them even and rhythmic by making each the same count (e.g. if you inhale to a count of 4, then hold 4 and exhale 4). As you improve, make the hold and exhalation longer and slower until the ratio is 1:4:2 (inhale 1: hold 4: exhale 2). For example, if you inhale to a count of 4, then hold 16 and exhale 8.

5. Begin by practicing for about 5 minutes at a time. Gradually increase until you are able to continue to do Alternate Nostril Breathing for 20 minutes without rest. If you find yourself running out of breath, you need to exhale more completely each time. Soon, you will be able to maintain the proper breathing ratio without counting.

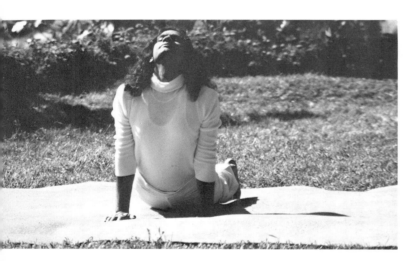

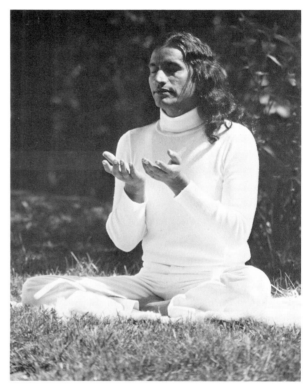

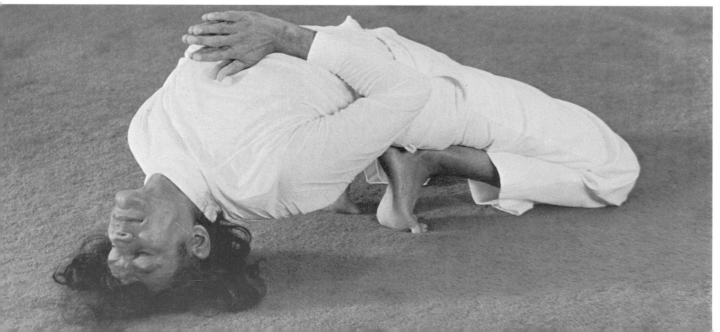

KRIPALU YOGA

The Yoga Especially for Westerners

Kripalu Yoga is a totally new approach to yoga developed especially for modern Westerners by Yogi Amrit Desai. He first set down its basic elements 10 years ago, although it is the fruit of a lifetime's deep experience of yoga. Since 1970, he has been developing, refining and testing these original concepts. The complete five-stage technique will soon be available to the public in his new book, *Kripalu Yoga*.

What makes Kripalu Yoga unique is that it is personally tailored to the needs of each individual. How? Through prana. It starts with the conscious, mentally-directed, disciplined practice of specific postures, as does traditional Hatha Yoga. Where it differs is in the method of progress. In traditional Hatha Yoga, the student concentrates on two things: (1) learning to come closer and closer to the "perfect" or ideal way of performing the posture, as pre-determined, perhaps arbitrarily, many centuries ago; and (2) learning an ever-widening variety of postures of increasing difficulty to challenge the body's limits more and more. There is often great effort involved and sometimes straining of the body, as we decide in our minds "I *will* do this", or "I *should* be able to do this."

Yoga, Prana and You

Progress in Kripalu Yoga comes through learning to be more and more in touch with the messages of prana in the body so that the postures begin to emerge as spontaneous movements responding to what prana knows the body needs. Prana's function is always to re-establish and maintain homeostasis -- balanced functioning of the whole organism; body, mind and spirit. Kripalu Yoga is thus a holistic approach to yoga from the beginning. (Of course, the ultimate goal of all yoga, as we saw, is holism.)

It is because Kripalu Yoga emphasizes development through learning to let prana move the body as it needs that it can be such a personally-tailored growth technique. No external source can tell us exactly what we need in terms of bodily exercise, the way that our prana, our own inner source of evolutionary energy, can. Kripalu Yoga takes yoga back to its ancient origins as spontaneous movements happening to advanced yogis in deep states of meditation, and only much later formulated into specific "postures". The movements that occur during advanced Kripalu Yoga may not even look like traditional "postures". In fact, they are the precursors of postures, pranic movements.

Kripalu Yoga is thus a more personal and pleasurable way to experience yoga. It is pleasurable because whenever we are attuned to prana we feel a deep sense of peace and well-being.

Yogi Desai has formulated it into five graduated stages, starting with traditional learning of the posture and culminating in the ecstatic experience of a spontaneous "posture flow", an organically interconnected series of movements performed automatically by prana with the mind merely playing the role of witness.

Even in the very early stages, Kripalu Yoga is practiced in a way that makes it unique, because it is a constant experience of getting in touch with prana. The whole secret is in coordination of breath with movement, because breath is the major carrier of prana.

Spontaneous and Absorbing Meditation

Here is what you would experience if you were in a Kripalu Yoga class. You begin to learn pranayama, as in most traditional yoga classes, but the difference is that you practice yogic deep breathing *as* you are doing the postures, and you do the postures very slowly with your eyes closed. As you are actually performing a posture, you learn to synchronize every movement with a deep, long yogic inhalation or exhalation. In a way that is almost miraculous, you are quickly drawn into a meditative state of great inner peace and mental quiet. When the eyes are closed, the combination of slow, regular, deep breathing; sound in the back of the throat; and very slow, flowing movements, has an effect upon your mind that is totally absorbing. You become fascinated by experiencing the extremely slow movements, and the sound of your own breathing is like a lullaby or like the sound of the mother's heartbeat to the baby in the womb.

Kripalu Yoga: Dance or Prayer?

Kripalu Yoga is something that has to be experienced to be understood. At the end of this chapter, you will find a "How to" section which will guide you through some Kripalu Yoga Meditation-in-Motion experiences. To help you visualize what it is like, try to see, in your mind's eye, an outstanding ballet dancer moving underwater. Every move has an energy, a beauty, a precision, yet it also has the dreamlike qualities of underwater movement. It is elegant, flowing, ultra-slow, constantly moving. One position flows endlessly into another, without interruption. until it becomes impossible to say where one ends and another begins. Yoga is no longer a series of exercises and static postures. It becomes an exquisite dance. When the body moves in this way, the inner experience reflects the external beauty and the whole activity begins to feel like a meditation, like a prayer -- an expression of the inner beauty latent in us all. No matter how ungainly, clumsy, or ungraceful anyone usually feels, in the Kripalu posture flow, everyone looks beautiful, as our pictures show. It is a truly amazing experience. This grace and beauty happens immediately, for although you can go on perfecting Kripalu Yoga for the rest of your life, even as a beginner you will have an immediate experience of physical grace, of inner beauty.

The Five Stages of Kripalu Yoga

The five stages into which Kripalu Yoga has been systematized by Yogi Amrit Desai each highlight a particular aspect of the practice. They correspond to the classical 8 stages of the complete practice of Hatha and Raja Yogas delineated by Patanjali in his *Yoga Sutras*. Yet while those 8 stages are practiced sequentially in classical yoga, in Kripalu Yoga they are experienced simultaneously. Although each stage focuses on one aspect of the discipline and is a pre-requisite to the stage that follows, foretastes of the more advanced stages will be experienced from time to time at the earlier levels, so that you are unlikely to get bored or impatient waiting to "get there," to experience the perfected skill. This is another thing that makes Kripalu Yoga unique.

STAGE ONE - MASTERING THE POSTURE. At this level, you simply learn the correct way to do the postures, doing them at your own comfort level (although, of course, you go on *perfecting* the posture for many years, as the body becomes more flexible).

STAGE TWO - CO-ORDINATING THE BREATHING WITH THE POSTURE. Here, the focus is on synchronizing the deep yogic breathing with every movement -- inhaling as you unfold and stretch, exhaling as you bend over or curl up.

STAGE THREE - HOLDING AND CONCENTRATING. In this stage, you learn to move even more slowly and to remain in the posture for a period of time, while *concentrating the energy of your attention* on the part of the body particularly affected by that posture.

STAGE FOUR - CREATIVE VISUALIZATION AND AFFIRMATION. In this stage, you learn to consciously *direct your inner energies* (prana) to the part of the body being benefitted by the posture, and to deliberately and willfully increase the benefits by visualizing relaxation and healing energy in the form of light and heat flowing to that area.

STAGE FIVE - SPONTANEOUS POSTURE FLOW. The purpose of the preceding 4 stages of mental and physical discipline is to help you get more in touch with your prana and to facilitate its free flow through your body. Next, you progress to the point where you cease to direct your movements with your mind, allowing them to become spontaneous and unchoreographed. At this point, prana itself is allowed to take over, while the mind simply becomes a witness to what happens. Earlier the mind was learning to become an agent of prana, rather than of the conscious, individualized ego. Now the mind is gently set aside as the inner wisdom of the universal life force directs the movements of your body, just as it does with a newborn baby or a cat stretching after sleep.

The Benefits of Kripalu Yoga

What are the benefits of Kripalu Yoga? They are those of the whole of the Kripalu Approach to Holistic Health. The more you are able to attune to prana and to free its energy from mentally-imposed blocks and conditions, the more it will heal and rejuvenate your body. You become progressively more relaxed, healthy, and in tune with life, with your true inner being, with those around you. You will feel more graceful, vibrant and whole -- in a word, more alive. You will find people are drawn to you because being with you makes them feel that way too, and you will increasingly enjoy being with yourself.

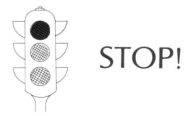

STOP! How aware are you of your body's messages *right now?* How are you feeling? Is there tension, stiffness, tiredness in any part of your body? Do you need to get up and stretch? Take some deep breaths? Relax your shoulders? Rest your eyes? Rest your mind? Close your eyes for a minute and take some long, slow deep breaths to enable you to get in touch with your experience. Then respond to what your body is asking you to do.

Taking a Posture Through the Five Stages

STAGE 1: PERFECTING THE POSTURE

STAGE 2: BREATH AND MOVEMENT COORDINATION

Note: We've combined Stages 1 & 2 of Kripalu Yoga in these directions for easy following.

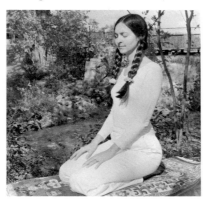

1. To begin, kneel with palms down on your thighs. Sit straight, but relaxed. Close your eyes. Take slow, deep breaths through the nose, breathing into the abdomen fully. Take a moment to relax. Concentrate your attention and energy on your body.

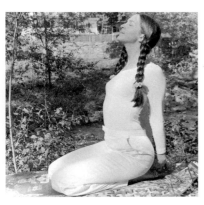

2. Inhaling slowly, raise your hands up from the thighs, and let them float very slowly around behind your hips. Imagine that the inhaled breath is moving them through space.

3. Holding the breath for a moment, interlock your fingers, pull the shoulder blades together, and drop the head slightly back.

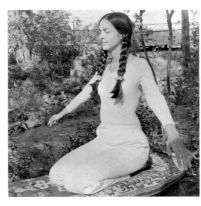

4. Gently exhale, very slowly. While exhaling, begin to bend forward, raising your arms and interlocked hands over your head. Bend forward until your forehead or chin rests on the floor.

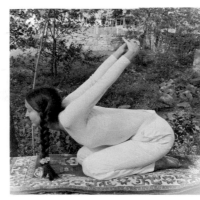

5. Breathe slowly and deeply using Yogic Deep Breathing while holding. Hold as is comfortable for you -- in the beginning, this may be a very short time. Do not strain.

6. As you gently inhale, rise SLOWLY up again, leading with your arms. Rise until your head is erect, your hands behind your hips. Keep shoulders relaxed, not hunched.

7. Exhaling fully, lightly release the fingers and let the arms float on the exhaling breath back to your thighs. Rest for a moment, still taking slow, yogic breaths, and feel the effects of the Yoga Mudra in your body and state of mind.

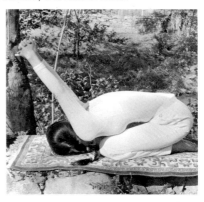

STAGE 3: HOLDING & CONCENTRATION

Close your eyes; become still and calm. Visualize yourself from this place of stillness moving effortlessly through the posture. Then repeat the Yoga Mudra as guided in Stages 1 and 2. The mind is focused, absorbed in the body's movement. Try to increase your holding time in the bending forward position. Guideline: 5-10 seconds in the beginning, gradually increasing time to 3 minutes duration. As you hold the position, continue with slow, deep yogic breaths. Let yourself be absorbed in the holding and allow the posture to happen; do not strain or force.

STAGE 4: CREATIVE AFFIRMATION & VISUALIZATION

Still coordinating breath with movement, activate the life energy or "prana" within yourself through this stage of creative visualization. Read the following visualization to yourself several times. Then practice the Yoga Mudra and carry the visualization into your experience.

Gently and slowly, begin to move through the Yoga Mudra. As your arms and body move, feel that they are moving not through your conscious will, but through the rhythm and power of your breath. Imagine that you are moving under water, slowly, gracefully and silently. While you hold the posture, feel a deep peace descend over your mind and body. Watch the overstimulated, misused nerves and organs of your abdomen relax. Feel their gratitude for this welcome release from tension. Complete the posture with calm resolve to carry this physical and mental tranquility through your day's activities.

STAGE 5: INCORPORATING THE POSTURE IN A SPONTANEOUS FLOW

HOW TO PRACTICE MEDITATION-IN-MOTION

A Beginning Exercise

Before you begin to do a Kripalu Yoga posture flow, try this very simple exercise. It is so easy that anyone of any age or physical condition can do it, and do it well. Yet simple though it is, it will give you a deep and real experience of Kripalu Yoga. It will take you about 10 minutes:

1. Choose a quiet, secluded place and dim the lights. Begin by sitting in a cross-legged position on the floor (or if this is really uncomfortable, sit in a straight-backed chair with your feet on the floor in front of you). Keep your spine straight and hold your neck and back in alignment, chin parallel to floor and tucked in slightly. Close your eyes and relax your body.

2. Slowly rotate your head in both directions to release any neck tension. Shrug your shoulders a few times and rotate them up and back. Then, in order to release any tension in your hands and arms, make a fist with both hands and squeeze as hard as you can. Hold for a moment and then relax the hands. Shake the hands and fingers as if something was stuck on the ends of your fingers and you wanted to shake it off. Then allow your hands to relax as you place them on your knees, palms facing upward.

3. Begin to take long, slow, deep and uniform yogic breaths. Allow the deep breaths to relax your body and calm your mind even more.

4. After several minutes of breathing, focus your attention on the solar plexus. Visualize the pranic energy as a warm, luminous, liquid light glowing in the solar plexus. See it or feel it clearly.

5. Begin to picture the energy flowing up through the chest, down the arms and into the hands. Concentrate on directing all of the energy into the hands. Actually visualize the hands and fingers filling with light.

6. Continue to concentrate on the energy flowing into your hands until you feel them wanting to rise up from your knees. Allow this to happen. If your hands remain on your lap, you can consciously lift them gently off your knees and then allow the movement to continue on its own. Do not expect anything specific to happen. The key to this exercise is to concentrate on your own prana and *observe* its working. Let your hands continue to float upward, keeping your elbows at your sides. Let your hands move upward toward your face in an extremely slow -- almost invisible -- movement. You may feel your hands are being moved without your conscious will, and that is a real experience of prana.

As your hands approach your face, allow your fingers to move gently across your face according to the patterns which arise spontaneously from within. As the fingertips move across the face, they discharge prana, relaxing deep muscles and erasing lines.

7. Now allow your hands to drift back down to their original position, letting the movement be extremely slow, almost invisible. When the hands have come to rest on the knees, remain in a sitting position with your eyes closed for as long as you wish. When you are ready, gently open the eyes and allow the muscles of the body to stretch. Experience the rejuvenation, the healing that has happened within you.

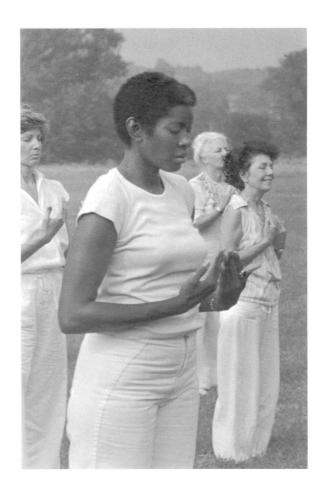

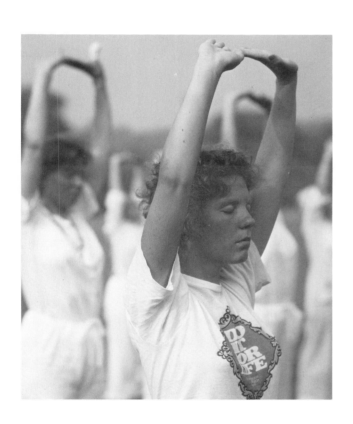

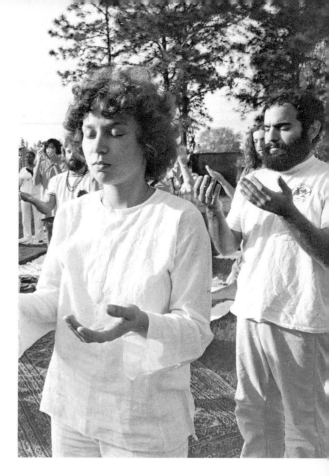

HOW TO DO A KRIPALU YOGA POSTURE FLOW

Although a spontaneous posture flow is the culmination of Krpalu Yoga practice in Stage Five, it is possible to experience a partially-spontaneous flow even at the beginning. The difference will be that you will not, at an early stage, experience your body as being completely guided by prana. Rather, you will experience your mind controlling your postures, yet allowing suggestions from prana to slowly come through. A pre-planned posture flow such as the one we suggest here is a way to begin to experience, through breath combined with movement, the sense of flow which will eventually connect you to your prana.

You can try this flow after a few months of practicing the postures of which it is composed. Wait until you have become comfortable with them, and can perform them without strain.

ALL MOVEMENTS SHOULD BE EXTREMELY SLOW, ACCOMPANIED BY DEEP YOGIC BREATHING. EYES SHOULD BE CLOSED.

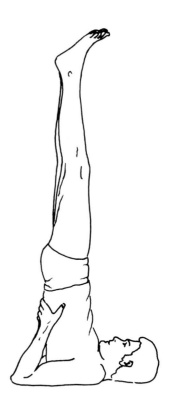

Step Two, Shoulderstand. Inhaling and moving very slowly, with eyes closed, come up into the Shoulderstand. Make no jerky movements, simply flow in a slow, relaxed manner. Be sensitive to every muscle movement, every articulation of a joint. Feel your body from the inside. Breathe deeply.

Step One, Relaxation: Lie on your back and become thoroughly relaxed by doing deep, rhythmic yogic breathing. It is very important to maintain this breathing throughout. It is your link with prana and should not be broken. Breathe in coordination with the component movements of the postures, as taught earlier in this section.

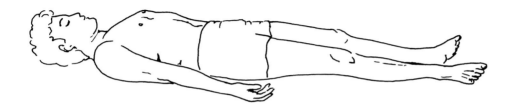

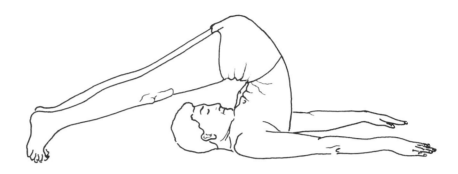

Step Three, Plough. After a slight pause in the Shoulderstand, begin to exhale and to slowly, very slowly, lower your straightened legs over your head until they come to rest in the Plough position. Breathe deeply.

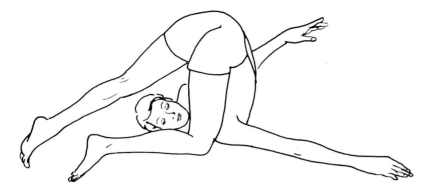

Step Four, Switchover. Exhaling, bring both legs to one side of the head, bending the inside knee and keeping the outside leg straight at first. Slowly roll over, bending the other knee, in a slow reverse somersault, ending up kneeling and seated on your heels. Breathe deeply.

Step Five, Camel. As you straighten up, very gently continue on back into the Camel. Do not bend back too rapidly or too far; you may lose balance or become dizzy. Breathe deeply.

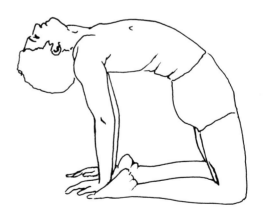

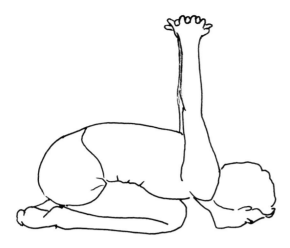

Step Six, Yoga Mudra. Exhaling, slowly come forward into the Yoga Mudra, clasping the hands as you come out of the Camel. Breathe deeply.

Step Seven, Relaxation: Come out of the Yoga Mudra into a relaxed kneeling or seated position. Breathe deeply and experience the internal effects. Become very aware of the deep sense of peace you feel as a result of your total absorption in your movements.

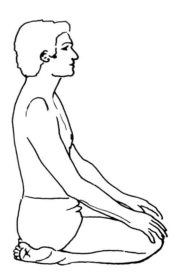

After some experience of different yoga postures, experiment with creating your own flow by holding each posture until your body signals what it wants to do next. After a period of time, you will begin to experience spontaneous movements and postures, or perhaps just stretches, as your prana becomes activated.

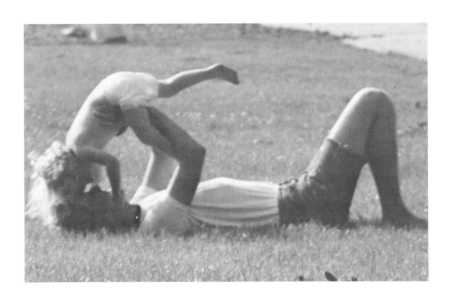

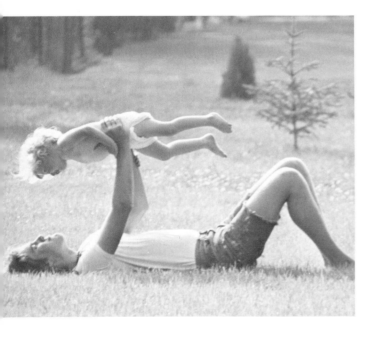

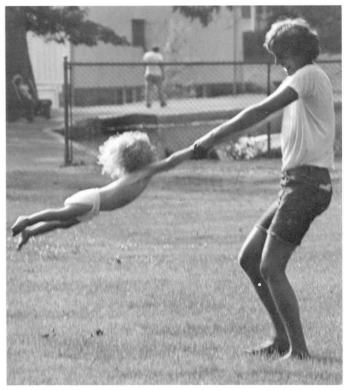

Self–Discovery Experience 8

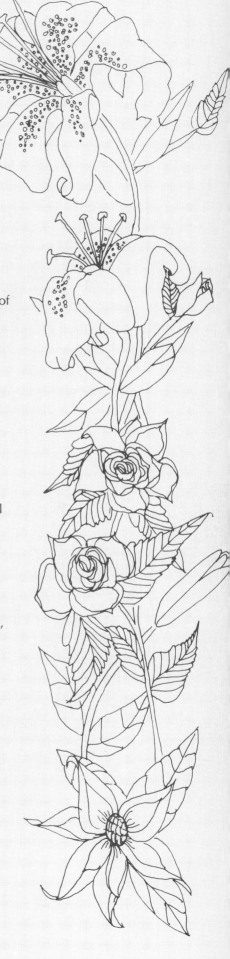

Rediscovering the Past Through Your Body

Awareness

After reading these instructions, close your eyes and relax, allowing the answers to come to you spontaneously from the feelings in your body rather than from the thoughts in your mind. Let this be an experiential trip into the past for you.

1. Going over your whole body, part by part, try to get in touch with its personal history. Recall incidents in the past that particularly involved that part of your body. It might be a time when you were injured, or when you became especially conscious of how much you depended on it. For example, you might get in touch with the time or times that you fell off your bike as a child and grazed your knee. Or the time you broke your wrist, had your arm in a cast and couldn't do the things you wanted to do. Really get in touch with how you felt at that time.

2. Also remember the times when a particular part of your body pleased you or surprised you. For instance, recall how good you felt about your legs one day when you ran a race faster than ever before, or when someone complimented you on your healthy feet or good posture.

3. Jot down for yourself, as you go, the words and images that come to you, or make drawings if that feels more appropriate.

Acceptance

What have you learned about your body that you didn't know before? Write down all the thoughts, feelings and emotions that came to you as you did this exercise.

Adjustment

Write down some specific things that you see you can or need to do to benefit from what you have just become aware of and what you have learned. For example, you might realize that you need to work at making your arms and shoulders more flexible, after remembering a time when you learned to hold them rigidly as a result of an experience that had a profound impact on you.

JOGGING & RUNNING

1. Why Run?

Modern medicine has compiled an impressive list of physical benefits that come from daily exercise, especially from swimming, wrestling and running or jogging. Of these three, running is by far the most frequently and most conveniently practiced, and its benefits are dramatic on the mental and emotional as well as the physical level.

The physical benefits of jogging and running are many. Your body will soon begin to lose excess weight. Your muscles become compact and toned all over your body. Your skin tightens and takes on a rosy glow of health. Your capacity for work of all kinds is increased. Your movements become quicker, more energetic and fluid.

By stabilizing and physically purifying the body through running, your emotions also become more stable and less subject to reaction and irritation. Through focusing on the physical realities of running, your mind becomes more steady and less restless. Jogging, and even more so, running (especially longer distance running) can become a wonderful means to forget the everyday cares of the world as you become focused on the body, the fresh air and the beautiful scenery.

2. Who Should -- and Shouldn't -- Jog or Run

Running is not a difficult sport, but there are a few beginning awarenesses that may save you physical discomfort and discouragement as you begin your running program.

If you are out of condition, over 35, or have a specific physical problem that may be affected by running, a medical check-up should be your first step. If possible, select a doctor who is also a runner, or at least, is somewhat sympathetic to its benefits. Some conditions that may warrant special medical guidance in jogging or running are: advanced arthritis, heart disease and hypertension, some orthopedic problems, and diabetes. Men over 35 should have check-ups even if they feel they are in good health and physical condition. A stress electrocardiogram (measuring the heart's reaction to physical effort) is recommended by many running experts and doctors.

Some physical conditions, such as those involving the heart, may be improved through a sensible program of jogging, but this should never be attempted without a doctor's supervision.

3. How Do I Start?

If you are out of condition, begin gradually and gently, with jogging rather than running (which is faster and more demanding). Remember how long it took for you to get into that condition and accept the fact that you cannot change it overnight. Begin by practicing some stretching exercises each day (the yoga postures described in this book would be an excellent place to begin), followed by a brisk walk. When you find you can walk for 15-20 minutes without tiring, add intervals of slow jogging to your walk. Jog slowly and gently until you feel yourself begin to tire or strain, then walk until you are ready to jog again. Repeat these intervals of jogging and walking as often as you can with comfort. Gradually your intervals of jogging will increase and, in time, the need to walk will disappear.

Do not worry about the distance you cover, especially if you are a beginner. If you need a challenge, set a length of time, rather than a distance, to remain out (20-30 minutes is a good beginning) and gradually increase it as you feel able. However, do not push yourself too far, too fast -- it should be enjoyable. To see whether or not you are pushing, check if you can hold a conversation as you run. If you get too out of breath, you need to slow down!

4. The Microcosm of Running -- A Personal Experience

Easily moving through space, through a gentle countryside, feeling revitalizing cool air pouring in and out -- I'm running with me. Like many runners, I have always experienced a peaceful and deep sense of myself during a run. But my experience with yoga has brought new and deeper benefits. When I run I gain deeper knowledge and insight into my inner world. I can see only too clearly my overall attitudes mirrored in my reactions towards hills, barking dogs, rainstorms and sunrises. Everything becomes so symbolic.

When my mind hits a "snag" while running, I can feel the tension immediately because it makes my breath laborious and I lose freedom of movement. And when I'm 4 or 5 miles from home, I have no choice but to deal with whatever is inside of me, then drop it by the wayside. I've realized more and more that what I see as problems must really be very insignificant if I can drop them so easily!

There's no overlooking the numerous physical benefits of running. But more importantly, I've come to see that by coming in touch with true joy at least once a day, my whole life has just naturally changed for the better.

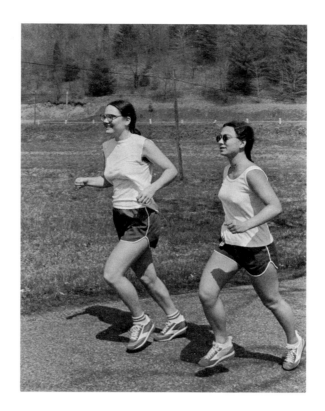

Joy creates a thirst for more, which has made me aware of my diet and use of energy. I can feel the benefits of proper eating so clearly each morning as I head off over the hills.

Lastly, I've seen that the happier my body is, the happier my mind is, and the happier my spirit is -- an amazing cycle that wonderfully feeds and perpetuates itself.

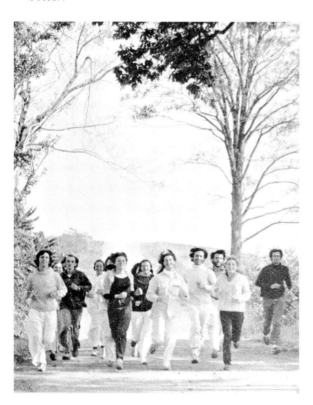

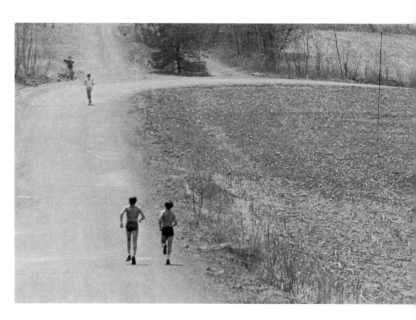

5.Some Kripalu Hints on Jogging and Running

Two things which the Kripalu Approach emphasizes when you run or jog are to always be gentle with yourself and never strain or force it; and to make it an internal experience of yourself and your body, not a competition or a test of endurance.

Always give your body time to warm up at the beginning of a jog or run by starting slowly. This will allow the blood vessels to expand, the blood to circulate more freely, and enough oxygen to be carried to the muscles for aerobic combustion (burning blood sugar for fuel in the presence of oxygen). Starting too fast causes anaerobic (without oxygen) combustion which builds up toxic wastes in the muscles, such as ptomaine and lactic acid. This results in pain and strain. Some anaerobic or "resistance" running is beneficial for accelerated burning of fat and strengthening of muscles but it should be done only after the body is thoroughly warmed up. Anaerobic running means running without burning oxygen in the cells, and is thus more demanding on the organism.

Concentrate on your breathing, making it deep and regular -- it will carry you along.

Focus your attention more on your own body awareness and inner experience, rather than on how far or how fast you can run.

Do it regularly -- with regular practice the body will get slimmer, firmer and more able to handle stress on all levels.

Do wind-down stretching exercises at the end for at least 5 minutes.

What Equipment Do I Need?

SHOES

Shoes are the only major purchase you will need to make to begin running -- and the most important. The proper shoes will save you needless discomfort and even injury, so take time to select them well.

Much has been written on the subject of choosing running shoes. A little research will yield a flood of valuable information. Then let your experience complete the process by visiting a number of stores and trying on a variety of brands and types. Be sure to wear the socks you plan to run in. Don't rush -- or let a salesperson rush you.

Check each pair for fit and comfort, light weight and flexibility. Are the soles durable, yet cushioned to absorb shock? Is there enough room for the toes and support for the heels?

CLOTHING

Expensive running outfits may be enjoyable if you can afford them, but they are not a necessity. Simple items of clothing that you may already own or which can be purchased inexpensively will suffice. What is important is comfort and suitability to the weather.

In hot weather, clothing should be minimal. Nylon is very popular for its light weight, but cotton will absorb perspiration and allow it to evaporate. Cotton also will not trap body heat. Light colors or white will reflect heat and a light cap will keep the sun from your head.

In cold weather do not dress too warmly. Allow for the body heat you will be generating. Layers of clothing will help to keep you warm, as the body heat warms the air between the layers. Also, you may want to remove a few layers as you get too hot (but be sure to put them back on as soon as you stop, or you will get chilled). A windbreaker (usually nylon is preferred) is very useful because it is lightweight but keeps in the body heat. A warm cap is also advisable, since 80% of the body's heat escapes through the head.

Most runners prefer socks in summer and winter to avoid blisters. Cotton or wool socks will absorb perspiration.

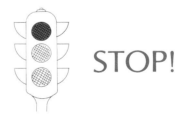

STOP! How aware are you of your body's messages *right now*? How are you feeling? Is there tension, stiffness, tiredness in any part of your body? Do you need to get up and stretch? Take some deep breaths? Relax your shoulders? Rest your eyes? Rest your mind? Close your eyes for a minute and take some long, slow deep breaths to enable you to get in touch with your experience. Then respond to what your body is asking you to do.

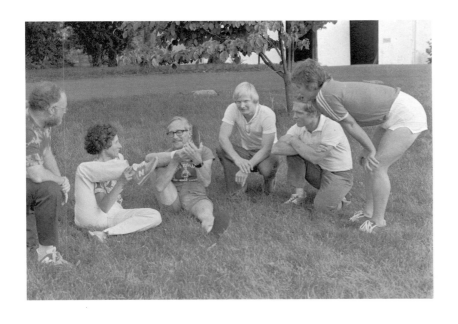

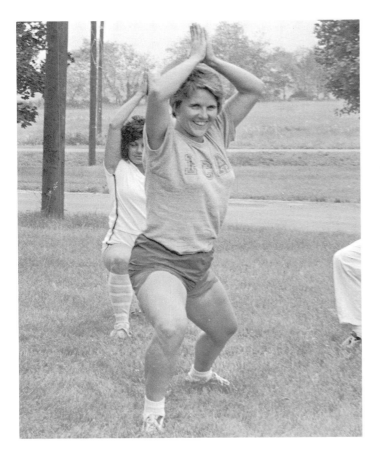

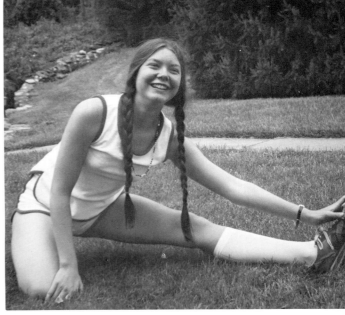

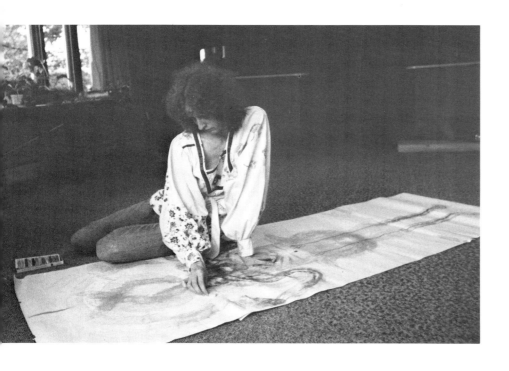

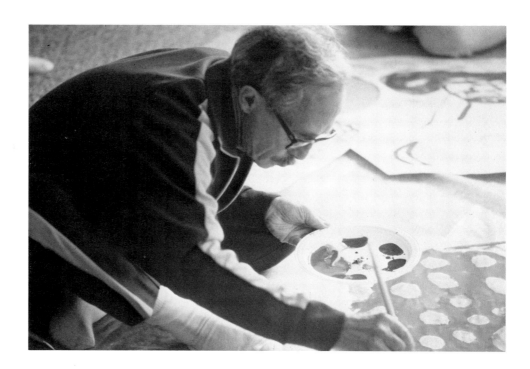

Self-Discovery Experience 9

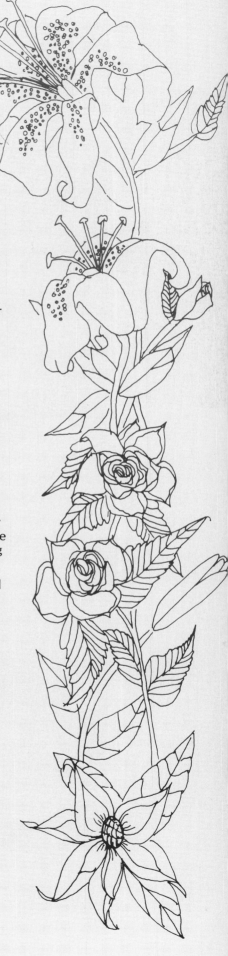

Body Mapping

Awareness

1. Sit quietly and come into touch with your body again. Be aware of how it feels to you; experience every minute inner movement, every change of pace. Begin to see your body in vivid colors. Give a color and shape to each part and organ, even if you do not know technically what it is, where it is or what it looks like. Use your creative imagination to visualize it.

2. Open your eyes, take some colored crayons and, without beginning to think too much about it, start to draw a map of your own body. Allow the map to illustrate your feelings about your body, as well as how you experience it in an objective way. For example, if you really like and feel good about one particular part of your body, try to draw/color in that feeling. If a part gives you trouble, see if you can depict that in some way.

Acceptance

1. Now take a long, hard look at your "map." See what it tells you about yourself and your body image and perceptions. Look at it very objectively, as if it was drawn by someone else. See what you can learn from it, in terms of what your unconscious thoughts are about your body, as opposed to the habitual way you think.

Adjustment

1. Now decide what this all implies for you. Is there some adjustment that you need to make in your image of yourself. Is there a disparity you'd like to remedy between what you consciously think of your body and your unconscious image of yourself? For example, do you see that you have drawn the top of your body out of proportion to the bottom? Does that perhaps mean that you need to pay more attention to what is going on in the lower part of your body?

2. Again, write some very specific ways you can work with what you have just learned about yourself that you didn't know before.

MASSAGE: A Helping Hand to Free Up Your Prana

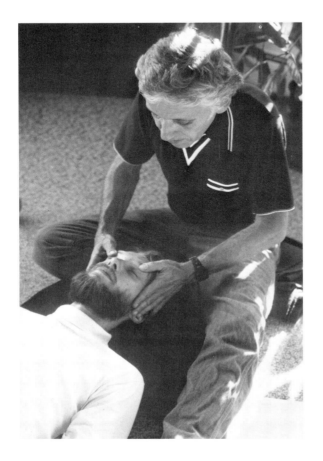

Massage is a time-honored method of relieving muscular distress. It was used by the ancient Greeks and Romans, and the Egyptians before them to relieve physical pain and injury and make the body supple. But it plays an even more fundamental role in Holistic Health. The Kripalu Approach teaches that physical tension and stiffness do not just stem from physical activity or inactivity. The body is actually a mirror reflecting our mind and emotions, so that physical tension is a result of what we are experiencing mentally and emotionally. Throughout our lives we are exposed to potentially tension-producing situations and this mental tension is expressed in our bodies. Because this is often unconscious, we do not take steps to dissipate the tension and it gradually builds up over the years. We generally experience tension in the same parts of our bodies habitually (neck and shoulders, forehead, lower back abdomen) and so, over a period of time, these patterns of tension become permanently lodged in our bodies as energy blocks, without our realizing it. Visualize the energy of water blocked by a twist in the garden hose . This affects our health, our posture, our mind and emotions, our whole way of being in the world. Tension thus inhibits our ability to experience the full freedom of body and mind which is the essence of Holistic Health.

The cornerstone of the Kripalu Approach to Holistic Health is, as we have seen, attuning ourselves to prana energy, and relaxation of physical and mental tension is a pre-requisite to this. Massage is a key way to get in touch with prana because it can dissipate tensions lodged in the muscles, not just in the preceding hours or days, but over a lifetime. Often during a massage recipients will re-experience a painful situation of many years before as they experience physical release of tension during the massage of a particular

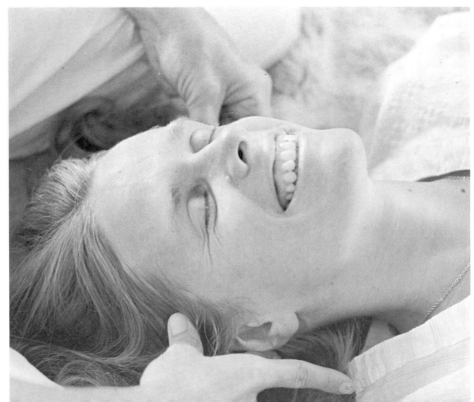

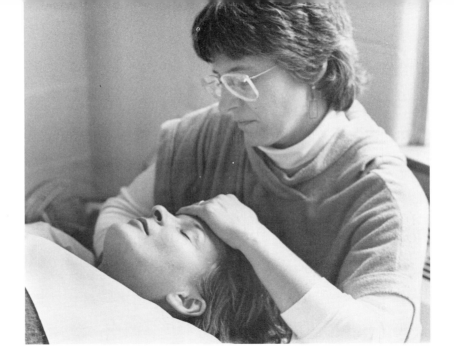

part of the body. They report that afterwards they feel sure they had been released from the stored emotional trauma as well as the physiological one.

Specific Therapeutic Benefits of Massage

In physiological terms, what happens in the course of a thorough, therapeutic, deep body massage is this:

- The circulation improves as the blood vessels dilate from the warmth of friction.
- Wastes and toxins are released and eliminated from the tense muscles by the pressure.
- Muscle tone is improved so the muscular system functions better.
- An increased flow of nutrients to the muscles is facilitated by the improved circulation and relaxation of the muscle fibers.
- Psychologically, people who receive a massage begin to enjoy their bodies more, to feel better about the body, as it feels better to them, and this positive attitude in turn produces greater health and vitality.

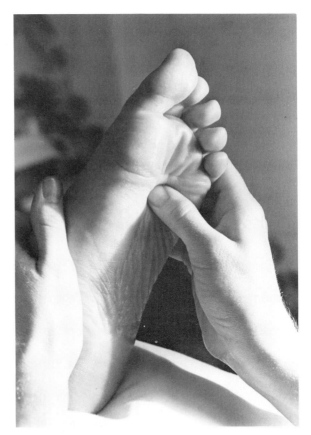

Massage as Meditation - A Personal Experience

"I had forgotten it was called a Meditation Massage. I was only expecting to have my body relieved of its aches and stiffness, to feel muscles unknot and joints loosen up, to be massaged into physical relaxation. And this certainly happened. But there was so much more. I didn't realize how totally lost I had become in the experience until I had to get up to use the bathroom in the middle of it. It was a tremendous effort to speak my need, to open my eyes, to get up and walk down the corridor. It was as if I were in another reality; everything looked strangely beautiful to me, as if I had forgotten where I was. That was the first clue. When I returned, I sank back immediately into the experience. Towards the end, I was conscious of my energy being pulled so strongly to the third eye point in my forehead -- as I so often fail to achieve in seated meditation -- that I was hardly aware of the rest of my body. As the massage ended, I found I had no desire to move. I had been drawn so deep within myself. I just lay there, in a warm, blissful, inward, meditative state, completely lost in the now moment. I was still aware of thoughts [many thoughts in fact] passing through my mind. But, somehow they were distant, unimportant, like a dimly-heard radio in the background.

I was vividly aware of the energy circulating like a fine golden rain in my body; a great feeling of alertness filled me, and yet, it was overlaid with a deep stillness. I was content just to be there, lying motionless in the gathering dusk that I momentarily sensed through my closed eyelids.

Finally, after a timeless span of experience, I shivered and became aware of the coldness that had spread through my limbs with the withdrawn energy. I noticed with amazement that nearly three-quarters of an hour had passed since the massage had ended. With difficulty I aroused myself; I walked as if in a dream to the sauna. Even more strongly than before, I had a sense of being in a separate reality. I sat silently, gazing through the dim, aromatic shadows at the other two bodies stretched out on the cedarwood benches, and for a few moments it was as if I'd never seen the human body before. I felt as if I was staring with the wide-eyed, inquiring look of a small child. I had no desire to speak; once warmed through, I only wanted to find my masseuse and hug her; and thank her for the deep experience, for the shared love, for giving so freely and teaching me to receive, for the gentle firmness of her touch and for the deeply meditative space she had entered and into which she had drawn me through her own concentration and inwardness.

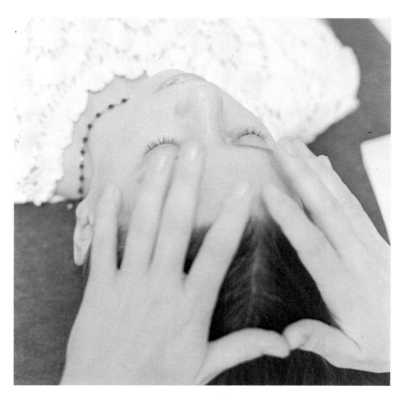

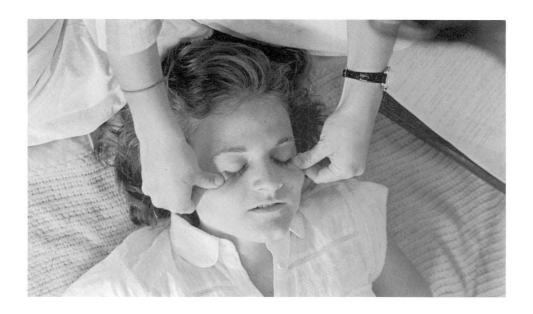

I tried afterwards to try to make conscious for myself the experience I had during the 1½-hour massage, which culminated in this deep, rare meditation. And it was not easy. These kinds of experiences are hard to conceptualize, let alone clothe in the poverty of language. In essence, I saw that it was an experience of being totally one with what was happening, one with my prana. After a few initial shared words of explanation and trust, my eyes had closed and I relaxed into just feeling. It is so rare for most of us to simply feel our bodies for an extended period of time, without judging, thinking, commenting. We have become so habituated to living in our heads, our thoughts and emotions. Only pain, very often, brings our consciousness back to the body -- and then with a sense of resistance and annoyance. Often, even in the sexual experience, there are so many other emotional and mental things going on -- the desire for pleasure, the fear of not giving satisfaction , the meaning of it all, the comparisons with another time, another place...

In this meditation massage, my mind was still, of course, active, but secondary, just a monotonous background voice that kept receding and fading. Effortlessly, my consciousness followed the firm, yet gentle fingers, discovering my body with them. I had been fasting and taking enemas, and had just had a sauna, so many of my customary pain and tension places [like neck and shoulders] were relatively loose and pain-free, to my surprise. But I discovered others, which amazed me. My legs felt fine until those probing fingers discovered the buried tensions and blocks in buttocks and thighs and calf muscles -- and the soles of the feet. Those strange reflex mirrors of the body felt like a burning iron was being run along them, yet it was only a thumb! And at these times, breathing deeply and slowly into the pain, as I have learned to do, I was astonished to see how far I have come in the past three years of Kripalu Yoga in dealing with pain. I don't fight it any more. I really know how to go with it; to ride its waves like a surfer; to embrace it and accept it as simply a part of my experience. And so pain has become transformed; no longer to be feared and fought. Not that the "pain" in a massage is like real pain from injury -- the acute sensation for which I have no other word than "pain" is really an exquisite suffering when it is releasing the other buried pain of tension and blockage.

The most amazing and beautiful thing in the massage was the pacing, the movement, the hands of the masseuse moved slowly and constantly across my muscles, always flowing at the same steady pace and pressure, always synchronized with an audible, deep breathing which in itself was deeply relaxing to hear, like the murmur of the tide on a distant seashore. This massage was indeed Kripalu Yoga Meditation-in-Motion, just as much as a Hatha Yoga posture flow, and thus had the same effect of drawing me into deep, effortless meditation. It was a unique and wonderful experience."

HOW TO GIVE A SIMPLE SHOULDER MASSAGE

The Prana Attitude:

Attitude is the key to the Kripalu method of massage. Anyone can learn the mechanics and physical moves of massage, but a truly loving, giving, meditative approach makes all the difference between mere physical relief and the deep sense of peace and well-being afforded by a Kripalu Prana Massage. The key points are:

• Begin with a relaxed and loving attitude yourself, secure in the knowledge that however little you may know intellectually about technique, your prana will flow from you to the recipient if you are relaxed and loving.

• Know that giving truly is receiving (after you give your first massage, this will be your own experience). Because your prana flows more freely when you are deeply concentrated on giving another a massage and because of the satisfaction you will feel at giving them the gift of relaxation, you too will feel deeply relaxed and energized.

• Really BE THERE for your friend. Your prana flows immediately to where your attention is, and so if you concentrate fully on your hands, the healing force of prana will work through them (you will feel them become very warm and tingling with prana energy as you work.)

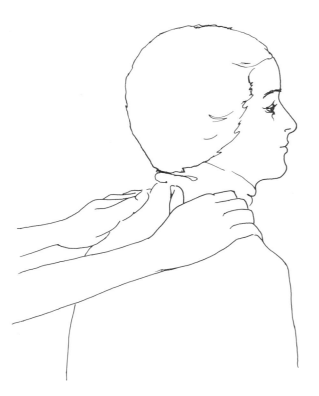

• Make the massage a meditative flow, a slow-motion dance. Breathe slowly and deeply, in harmony with your movements. As you become familiar with the movements, try working with your eyes closed.

• Visualize the prana as warmth, radiant liquid light flowing into the parts of the body you are massaging. Ask your friend to try to visualize it with you.

• Use firm, strong pressure. This communicates confidence and also feels better to the recipient. Keep your hands constantly touching his/her body, to keep the energy contact.

• Feel as if it is happening to your own body, so that you know exactly where and how to touch.

Step by Step Instructions

This simple neck and shoulder massage is most easily done with the recipient sitting on the floor, cross-legged or kneeling. Those with older or less flexible bodies may be more comfortable (and comfort is important for relaxation) sitting on a chair with their feet flat on the floor.

The massage has infinite variations -- let PRANA lead you! Draw on your own experience of what eases tension, and be guided by your inner sense of where tension is accumulated. Let your love flow!

1. Place your palms firmly on your friend's shoulders and make deep contact. Take a few deep breaths and ask him/her to do so as well.

2. Smooth down the arms and the entire back with light, gentle strokes. Use your whole hand.

3. Do a brisk circular rub with the heel of your hand down the whole of the back (divide the back mentally into vertical "sections" and do one at a time, top to bottom). Then rub the arms.

4. Shoulder Kneading - Keep your palm on the back of the shoulder as much as possible and "knead" the large muscle along the top of the shoulder by using your fingers (held together and "hooked" over in front of shoulder with care not to press directly on collar bone). Imagine you are kneading bread. Use the ball of your hand to push the muscle into the heel of your hand and thumb. The emphasis is on creating a smooth wave-like motion. Let your thumbs reach down between the shoulder blades to work that area, keeping your fingers still over the shoulders. Also let your thumb follow the curve of the shoulder blade, outlining the top and side closest to spine.

5. "Lift" the large shoulder muscle between your thumb and fingers. Press in and hold it briefly at tense spots, asking your friend to take deep breaths while you hold.

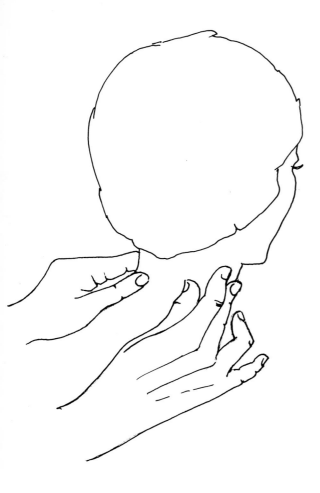

7. "Pinch" the muscles that run up either side of the spine at the neck between your thumb and first two fingers, working up the neck with a circling motion. This is very relaxing!

8. Do a light circling pressure along the ridge of the skull with thumb or fingers.

9. Press in and up with your thumb at the depression just under the ridge of the skull. Work a line from near the ear into just beside the spine on one side, then the other. Your friend can take deep breaths as you hold. This is particularly good for headaches.

10. Gently "slap" the head with both hands, starting at the center of the top and working all around.

11. Let the slapping motion flow down onto the shoulders and change to a "chopping" motion with sides of your hands, fingers loose (a gentle massage) or straight. Ask your friend to lean forward, and "chop" along the spinal muscles and back. Do this lightly also in the kidney area, just below the ribs.

12. Finish off by gently "smoothing down" the whole area you have massaged, by slowly sliding your hands several times over your friend from the crown of the head to the tips of the shoulders.

6. Use your thumbs to press directly down on the shoulder muscle in a line beginning at the "V" where the collar bone and shoulder blade meet at the outer edge of the shoulder, and working in toward the spine. There are points in this area which are VERY effective tension releasers. They are also likely to be very tender, so be gentle until you determine how hard to press. Good firm pressure is most effective. Ask your friend to take deep breaths while you hold these points. You will get better pressure if you "stand" on your knees. Ask for feedback as to whether you've found the right spot.

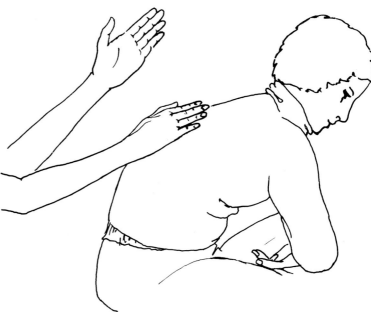

HOW TO GIVE YOURSELF A DO-IN SELF-MASSAGE

The Principles

Do-In is an ancient Oriental technique of self-massage which quickly relaxes and energizes the body by stimulating and harmonizing the flow of prana energy within the body (in the East called Chi or Ki). It is based on the same principles as acupuncture, which works with energy meridians (nerve channels which carry the energy of prana or Chi throughout the body) linking different organs. Thus, stimulating one point along a meridian will free the energy up and down the body along that channel. In Do-In (pronounced Doh-in) when one part of the body is massaged, the less accessible parts, including inner organs, are also being stimulated. (Foot reflexology is based on the same principle.) Do-In is a wonderfully fast way to get your energy moving when you wake up in the morning, as well as to release tension at the end of the day.

Step by Step Instructions

Take a comfortable position, preferably kneeling and sitting back on your heels. Relax and take some long, slow, deep breaths with your eyes closed and hands resting palms upward on your knees. When you feel calm and centered, you may begin.

Slowly stretch your arms up in the air above your head, extending the hands and fingers and tilting your head slightly back. Feel as if you are an empty cup, inviting the universal energy of prana to flow down into your being. Allow yourself to feel filled with energy before you start.

1. Head

Make loose fists with your hands and bring them slowly down to rest on the top of your head. Now begin to gently pound the top of your head, moving from the front to the back and from the center outwards, and finishing with the back of the neck. This is good for not only the head, but also the whole spine, the sinuses and, at center top, for hemorrhoids.

EARS

Gently pinch around the lobes of your ears with a rippling motion, starting at the top. Have your thumb on the front, fingers on the back. Then pinch and quickly pull your fingers away from three points: top, center and lower lobe. This is beneficial for both the kidneys and the intestines. Rub up and down in front of your ears with your index finger until you feel heat. This is good for the small intestines.

2. Face

FOREHEAD

Place one hand in the other, with the back of the right hand in the palm of the left, and bring them to rest lightly on your forehead. Keeping the hands still, gently turn your head from side to side so that it receives a gentle massage. Speed up slightly, then slow down again before stopping. This is very beneficial for the liver.

NOSE

Pinch the bridge of the nose firmly, hold for a few minutes, and then rub it. This is good for the sinuses and also the heart. Also pinch and massage your upper lip.

TEMPLES

Rub in a circular motion with three fingers to alleviate general tension.

EYES

With two fingers of each hand press gently all around the eyes, in a circle. Then cover them lightly with your palms for a short while and watch your inner sky.

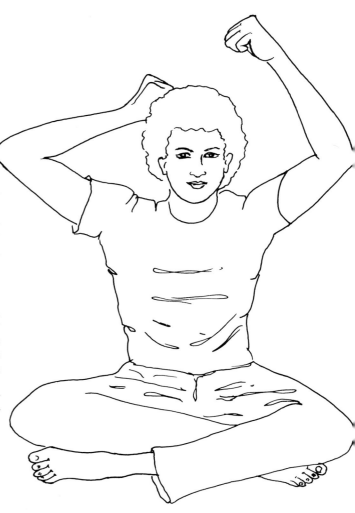

CHEEKS

Vibrate them with your palms to stimulate the lungs. Then tap vigorously with fingertips all along the cheekbones, starting at the nose, and moving out and down in front of the ears to the angle of the jaw. This is good for the large intestine, the sinuses, and also for depression.

JAW

With thumbs hooked under the jaw at its outside edge below the ear, and fingers on top, press in small circles towards the center. This helps relieve headaches and tension in the jaw, and is good for the gums and teeth.

MOUTH

Tap vigorously with the fingertips and massage, to benefit the gums and relieve tension. Stretch your mouth open and make noises. Move the jaw from side to side with your mouth wide open. This also facilitates release of tension.

PAUSE AND SHAKE OUT YOUR HANDS. FEEL AS IF YOU ARE SHAKING OFF TENSION AND EXCESS OR STATIC ENERGY. CLOSE YOUR EYES FOR A MOMENT AND FEEL THE PRANA CIRCULATING MORE FREELY IN YOUR HEAD AND FACE.

3. Upper Body

NECK AND SHOULDERS

With the right hand made into a loose fist, bring it across your chest and begin to pound vigorously down the left side of the neck and out to the tip of the shoulder. Support your right elbow in your left hand as you do this. Reach over to the back of your shoulder and pound the upper back muscle that you feel there. It holds a great deal of

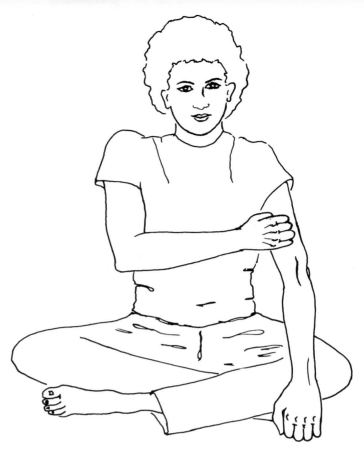

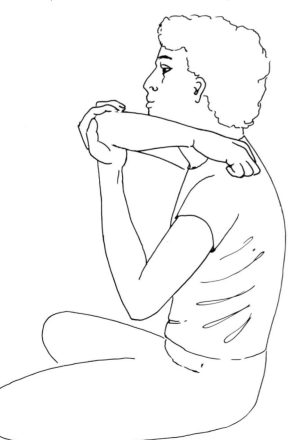

tension. Reverse hands and do the same for the right neck and shoulder. This stimulates the eliminative process, particularly in the large intestine.

ARMS

With your right hand made into a fist, pound down the inside of your left arm (to stimulate the heart and lungs) and then up the outside (to stimulate the large and small intestines, and to regulate body heat). Do this several times, then reverse arms.

CHEST

Pound the center of your upper chest at the start of your collarbone, moving out beneath it to your shoulders, and make a deep AAAHHHH sound as you do so, to release tension and to open up the lungs. This is particularly good if you have a cough.

Then pound down the center of your upper body and out along the bottom edges of your rib cage. Be more gentle here, as you are working with your liver, spleen and stomach.

INTESTINES

Gently pound your lower abdomen and pelvic area in clockwise circles (up the right side, across the top, and down the left) following the path of the colon.

PAUSE AGAIN TO SHAKE OUT YOUR HANDS AND TO FEEL THE ENERGY MOVING IN YOUR BODY, SITTING WITH EYES CLOSED FOR A MOMENT.

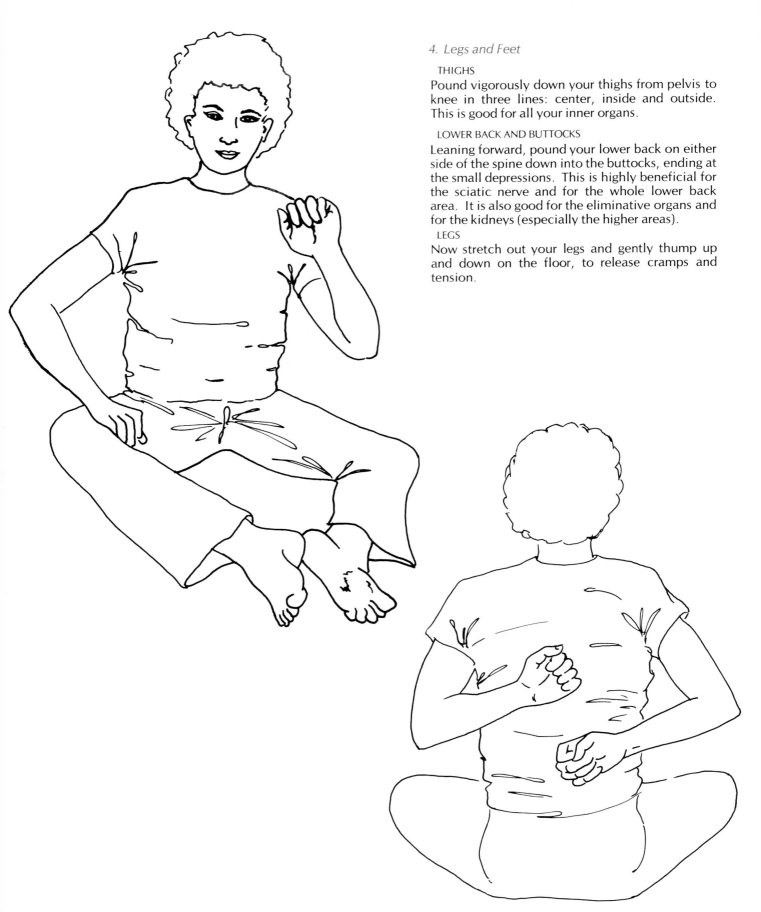

4. Legs and Feet

THIGHS

Pound vigorously down your thighs from pelvis to knee in three lines: center, inside and outside. This is good for all your inner organs.

LOWER BACK AND BUTTOCKS

Leaning forward, pound your lower back on either side of the spine down into the buttocks, ending at the small depressions. This is highly beneficial for the sciatic nerve and for the whole lower back area. It is also good for the eliminative organs and for the kidneys (especially the higher areas).

LEGS

Now stretch out your legs and gently thump up and down on the floor, to release cramps and tension.

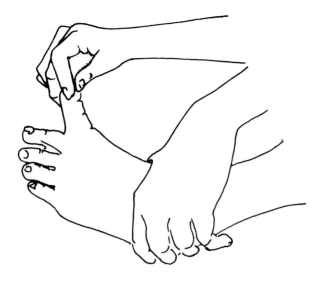

5. Hands

Finally, massage your hands, which have just done all this hard work! First, shake them out again to remove static energy and tiredness. Then, for each hand in turn, rotate and twist each finger with the whole of your other hand, bending it back and forth as you did with your toes. Crack your knuckles if you can, as this loosens the joints by re-distributing the sinovial fluid. Massage the palm of each hand with your fingers. This is good for the heart. Bite (gently!) the end of your little finger just to the outside of center near the top of the nail. This is also good for the heart and can, reportedly, even arrest a heart attack! Massage the webbed area between your thumb and first finger. Find, by probing deeply, the tender spot there and massage it deeply. There are pressure points here for the sinuses and the intestines, and massaging this area will help headaches, constipation and menstrual cramps. Shake out your hands one last time.

FEET

First with one foot and then the other, repeat the following motions. Lift your foot up with both hands, knee bent, and shake it out. Rotate your foot around your ankle while pinching the back of the ankle with the opposite hand to release any tension in ankle joint. Place your foot, sole up, on your opposite thigh and begin to pound vigorously up and down on the sole.

This stimulates your whole body, because the soles of the feet contain reflex points to all other organs of the body. Now press your thumbs one on top of the other for strength, in four lines from the heel to the toes along the sole of the foot. One line will follow the inside edge of the foot, two will be in the middle and the fourth will be along the very outside edge. Rotate the toes one by one, starting with the big toe. Then press each back towards the sole of the foot, and out towards the front of the leg before snapping your fingers sharply off the end of each toe.

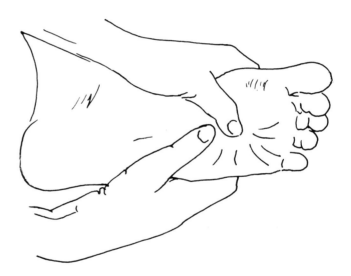

NOW SIT QUIETLY, WITH YOUR EYES CLOSED, AND BECOME SENSITIVE TO THE ENERGY NEWLY MOVING IN YOUR BODY. NOTICE EXACTLY HOW YOU FEEL DIF- FERENTLY THAN YOU DID BEFORE YOU STARTED. BE AWARE OF HOW YOU HAVE REFRESHED AND RE-ENER- GIZED YOUR WHOLE BODY BY THIS SIMPLE TECHNIQUE OF SELF-MASSAGE. PROMISE YOURSELF TO STOP AND DO IT WHENEVER YOU FEEL A BUILDUP OF TENSION AND TIREDNESS IN YOUR BODY.

OTHER HEALTH TOOLS

These facilities are offered at the Kripalu Center for Holistic Health, and we recommend them thoroughly if they are available in your area.

Sauna

A sauna uses heat to make the body perspire. Different processes for creating a super-hot environment to make the body sweat have been in use for thousands of years, even before the times of the Greeks and Romans, as a means to cleanse and purify the body. Many cultures throughout the world, from the Finns to the American Indians, have used equivalents of the sauna as an important technique for maintaining and enhancing health. Sauna itself, however, is a Finnish word (pronounced sow-na, in case you're interested) and institution.

What Happens to the Body During a Sauna?

Sauna uses heat to raise the outside temperature to anywhere from 180 degrees Fahrenheit to 225 degrees or more. Our bodies have a wonderful ability to adjust to such heat. The most important aspect of this ability is called sweat. There are 2 million tiny sweat glands situated just below the surface of our skin. Each one of these sweat

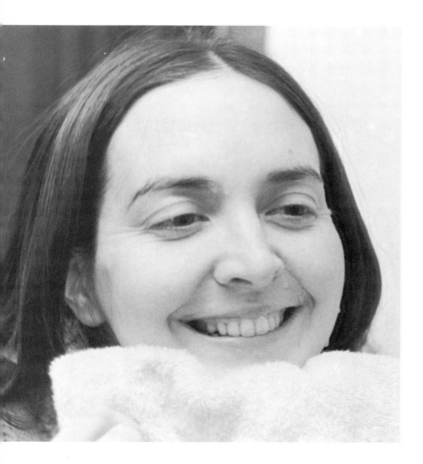

glands is a tiny coiled tube which is connected to our blood circulation system and is capable of bringing water to the surface of the skin through the tiny openings in the skin we call pores.

When the outside temperature increases, the blood circulation within the body also increases as a means of distributing the heat throughout the body. You will notice during sauna that your heart rate increases (sometimes up to 130 beats per minute; well above the norm of approximately 70 beats per minute). When the temperature increases to a certain point, the sweat glands begin to secrete a liquid which is almost pure water, but also contains some undesirable mineral wastes from the body.

Through the process of sweating and evaporation, the body machine is able to keep its inner temperature within a fairly constant range of 98 to 100 degrees Fahrenheit, even though the outside temperature is 180 degrees or more. You would appreciate your body's wisdom if you mistakenly wore your watch into the sauna. You would soon find that the metal on your watch had become too hot to touch. Metal doesn't sweat, but our skin does. This process of bodily heat control is another example of the workings of prana -- that innate inner intelligence of our body which works automatically, without the intervention of our conscious mind, to preserve and enhance our health.

What are the Benefits of Sauna?

1. *Bodily Cleanser & Beautifier:* In time, you'll have rosy skin as smooth as a baby's! All of the pores in your body will open wide and your whole skin will be cleansed from inside out (and the top layer of dead skin cells will be sloughed off). The increased blood flow gives your skin a healthful vitality and look of aliveness.

2. *Combats Illness:* During 15-30 minutes of sauna, your body can dispose of waste elements that would take your kidneys over 24 hours to eliminate. These accumulated waste elements in the body often lead to physical illness. Sauna helps to eliminate these wastes and thus make you healthier in body, mind and spirit.

3. *Relaxes the Body/Soothes the Nerves:* Sauna also provides a deep muscle relaxation for your body, as the increased circulation removes waste from tired muscles and nerves, allowing them to truly relax and rest.

How to Take a Sauna

The full sauna experience is a 3-step process of:

1) *heating up* to a sweat in the sauna
2) *cooling off* rapidly in a *cold* shower
3) returning to the sauna for *relaxation*

Experienced sauna-goers may repeat this process 3 or 4 times in one sauna session. You will remember that the benefit of sauna comes from increased blood circulation and sweating. This process of heating up and then cooling off rapidly tends to flush the inner organs with fresh blood, maximizing the benefits.

Sometimes people avoid the rapid cooling off because the cold water seems painful. This pain tends to disappear when you relax the body's muscles and breathe deeply in and out as the deliciously cool water stimulates the surface of the skin. For hours afterwards, people often feel a warm glow of heat that seems to come from deep within the body -- another experience of prana.

Another common sauna practice is to rub the surface of the skin with a loofa before and during the sauna; this is a dried gourd sponge which stimulates the blood circulation when rubbed on the skin. A natural bristle brush is also very effective.

Don't overdo your first sauna experience. Don't allow yourself to become dizzy with too much heat exposure. Most people find that 5-10 minutes is enough time in the sauna at first. Each person is different, so judge your own capacity. You may want to begin your first sauna by sitting on the lower bench where the temperature tends to be lower.

Who Should Not Take a Sauna

Those with medical problems, particularly those related to the heart or circulatory system, including hypertension and high or low blood pressure, should *consult a doctor* before taking a sauna, as it may not be advisable.

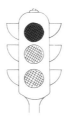

STOP!

STOP! How aware are you of your body's messages *right now?* How are you feeling? Is there tension, stiffness, tiredness in any part of your body? Do you need to get up and stretch? Take some deep breaths? Relax your shoulders? Rest your eyes? Rest your mind? Close your eyes for a minute and take some long, slow deep breaths to enable you to get in touch with your experience. Then respond to what your body is asking you to do.

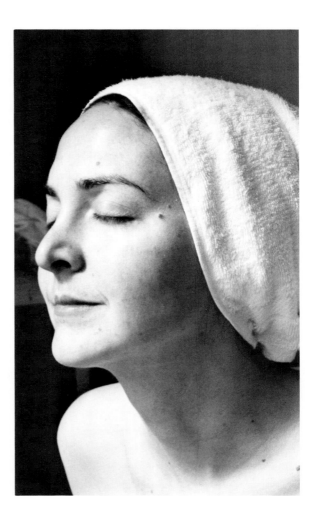

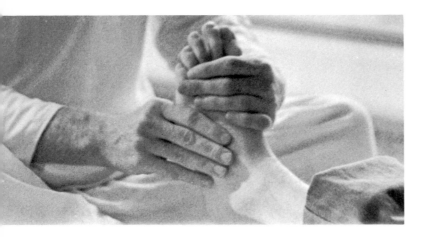

Reflexology is tremendously beneficial for those experiencing:

- constipation
- headache
- toothache
- tension
- backache
- shoulder pain
- indigestion
- overworked kidneys and gall bladder

Reflexology Foot Massage

Reflexology foot massage is an effective way to relax the whole body. All of the energy currents throughout the body flow through the feet. The foot, by virtue of its easy accessibility, is easily massaged, and as the pressure points in the feet are stimulated the corresponding organs and areas of the body experience stimulation and relaxation. The potency of reflexology is based upon the principle that every part of the body is reflexively connected with every other part. As the therapist locates and breaks up the crystalline salt deposits in the feet, the corresponding parts of the body are stimulated. This promotes the elimination of toxic wastes stored in the tissues that have been produced through incomplete metabolism. The musculature and fascia of the feet become supple and return to their original length and elasticity. After experiencing this "kriya" or yogic cleansing technique, people feel a heightened sense of being "grounded" and supported as they stand and walk.

Polarity Therapy

Polarity is the science of balancing the vital life force in the body, and is used to bring about deep healing relaxation. When the energy poles in the body are restored to their freely flowing equilibrium, a steady and peaceful feeling of health and well-being is experienced. Yogis have used these techniques spontaneously to realize high states of consciousness.

In a polarity session, gentle manipulations are used to direct the healing energy to specific areas in the body. The intelligent energy in the body is stimulated to break up physiological blocks and to restore the body's normal functioning.

The benefits of polarity are numerous, and extend to all persons, regardless of age or physical condition. They include:

- structural re-alignment and reduction of muscular and skeletal pain
- stimulation of all the vital organs and an energization of the glandular system
- an acceleration of the body's healing process promoted by the increase of available body energy

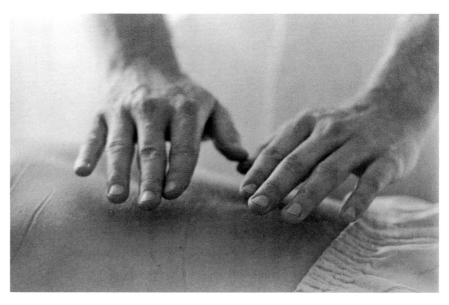

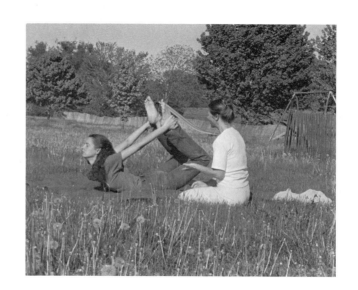

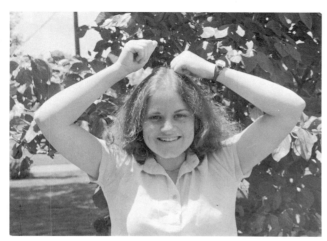

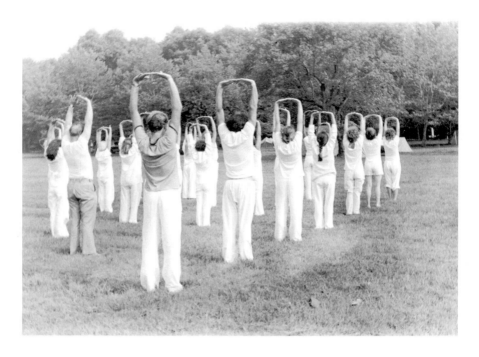

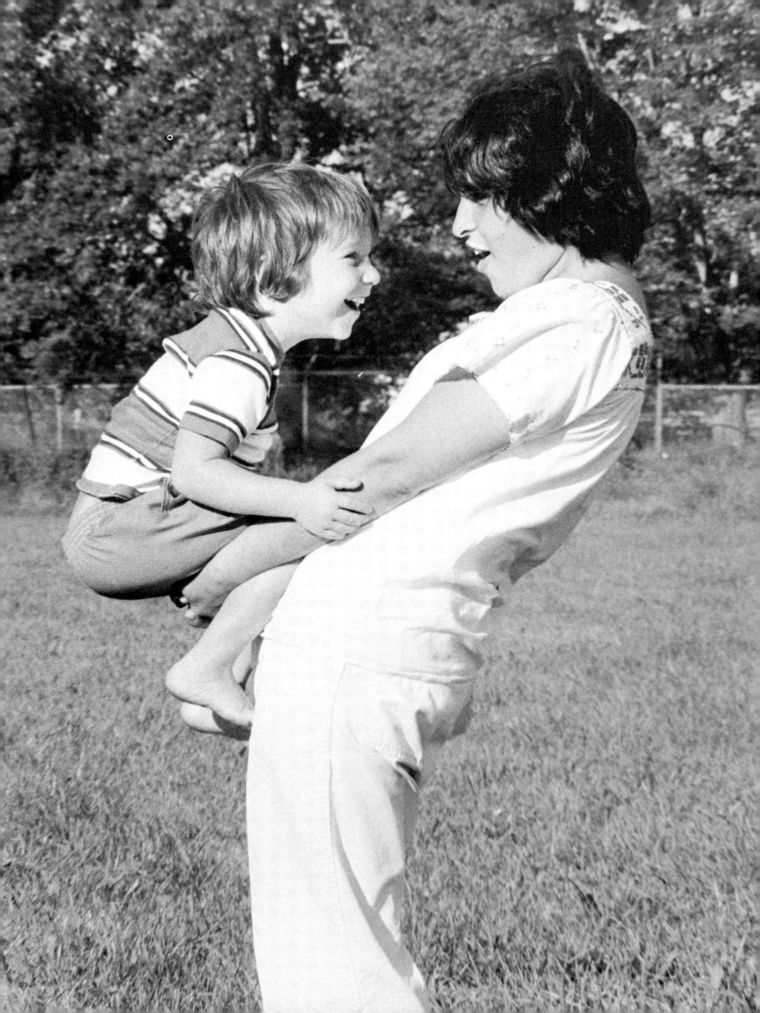

WAY THREE
learning how to play

The steps to Holistic Health that have been discussed so far are probably no surprise to you, but where does "learning to play" fit in? Play has become something that mature adults are not expected to do or take seriously. Sports, cultural activities, creative arts, studying -- these are praiseworthy and acceptable ways to spend the time when we are not working. But playing? Adults don't play, do they?

That is the whole problem. We seem to have come by the idea that any activity which has no goal (such as defeating an opponent) or tangible end result (such as winning a trophy) and does not demand concentration and brain power (such as chess or bridge) is not a valid way to spend time. We play with our children occasionally, but with each other? Hardly. Perhaps a party game or two, but we often feel rather foolish even then.

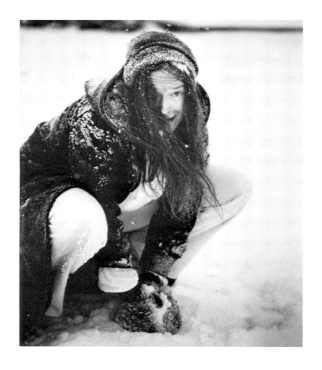

Yet play (light-hearted activity that has no apparent purpose) is an essential ingredient in Holistic Health, as are laughter and humor. If we enter fully into play, we lose ourselves in the fun of it. Then our minds and bodies relax as they become united in the activity. Laughter in itself is deeply relaxing because it loosens up the abdomen, releasing stress from the solar plexus, that storehouse of tension. Most of us take our lives far too seriously. If we could learn to laugh at our problems a little, to see the humor inherent in almost any situation, we would be more relaxed and thus healthier people. There is a child within us all who longs to be let out to play. Learning how to contact and enjoy that childlike aspect of ourselves is a vital part of the Kripalu Approach to Holistic Health.

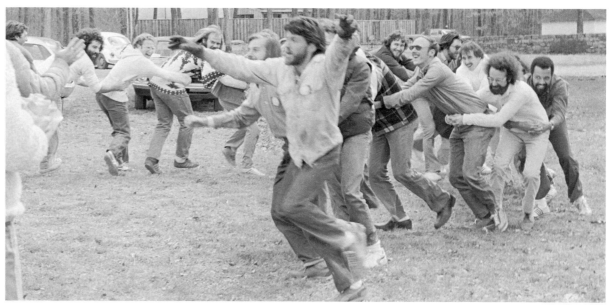

THE HEALING POWER OF LAUGHTER, PLAY AND HUMOR

"Good spirits are a vital part of life. Denying joy is one of the greatest deprivations on this planet!" So remarked Norman Cousins, Editor of *Saturday Review* and guest lecturer at UCLA Medical School. What is a journalist doing at a medical school? Teaching people how to heal with humor!

Cousins' expertise comes from his own direct experience. In 1964, he developed a serious collagen illness weakening the connective tissues of his body. His disease was diagnosed as progressively degenerative. After a toxic reaction to almost all the medication being given him in the hospital, Norman Cousins began to search for an alternative. He had read Hans Selye's *The Stress of Life* and began to question if perhaps his own emotions had played a hand in his illness. If so, could it be possible that positive emotions could create positive chemical changes in the body as well? "Is it possible that love, hope, laughter and the will to live have a therapeutic value?"

Cousins decided to test his hypothesis. In partnership with his physician, Dr. William Hitzig, he began a personal regimen that included, as a key part, activities designed to affirm positive emotions and use laughter as a healing force. It worked. Watching classics from the TV show "Candid Camera" was particularly effective. "I made the joyous discovery that ten minutes of genuine belly laughter had an anesthetic effect and would give me at least two hours of pain-free sleep." As time passed, continuing his new therapy, the connective tissue in his body began to regenerate. In the years since then he has resumed jogging, horseback riding and is almost pain-free.

In summarizing what he has learned, he says, "Never underestimate the capacity of the human mind and body to regenerate -- even when the prospects seem wretched. The life-force may be the least-understood force on earth. William James said that human beings tend to live too far within self-imposed limits. It is possible that those limits will recede when we respect more fully the natural drive of the human mind and body toward perfectibility and regeneration. Protecting and cherishing that natural drive may well represent the finest exercise of human freedom."*

How did the healing of Norman Cousins happen? Consider, for a moment, the last time you had a hearty belly laugh or played a good hard game of golf, baseball or even Monopoly! Where was your mind at the time? How did you feel emotionally? What was the experience of your body?

*Quotes and story from *New England Journal of Medicine,* December, 1976.

Laughter and Prana

If you consult your own experience, you'll most likely agree that play and humor are indeed "captivating." What do they "capture" us from? They save us from our reveries (and regrets) about the past and our hopes and anxieties about the future. Play and humor bring our mind into the moment, into here-and-nowness, into an almost sensuous experience of all that life is in that second. We become concentrated, but without effort. We become absorbed, but without tension. Through play and humor, prana, our inner-life force (the force Cousins called "the least understood...on earth") is freed to manifest and flow within us, unleashed from the blocks of mental control and physical inhibition. When we play and laugh hard, our prana is in "flow", is in harmony with the world and people around us. Free of roles, conflicting attitudes, social dictums, body and mind relax into "life", connecting with the life or pulse of prana around us. Energy is ignited rather than spent, creating an explosion of good feelings, positivity and connectedness.

Earlier, disease was defined as a condition wherein the flow of prana (the guiding intelligence of the body) has been blocked and chronically denied expression. In the experience of play or humor, we enter a world of ease, effortless freedom and faith. Mind, body and prana are harmonized. In this act of letting go, of celebration, prana is freed to do the work of healing.

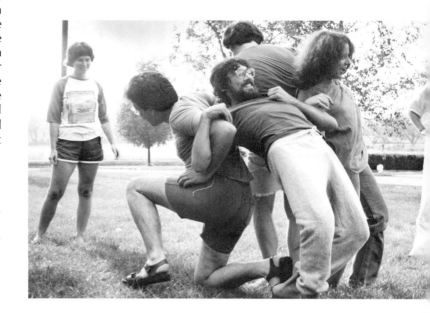

The Child Within

No one has to teach children how to play or laugh. They come into the world prepared to experience everything as if it were new; therefore, they are the first to be delighted at the simplest things.

Can you imagine a child thinking, "Gee, I haven't taken time to play this week; maybe I should plan an hour to have some fun...?" At the same time, have you ever known an adult who forgot to eat even once a day? So we all have priorities in life, some conscious and some unconscious. These priorities, nevertheless, have tremendous influence upon our lives.

Sadly enough, many of us, as we have grown up, have lost some of the innocent qualities we possessed as children. We've become too busy to take time to play. We're so caught up in the ambitious endeavor of making our dreams come true. Thus, we miss the joy and fun we were originally seeking.

Children make fun out of everything they do. A few pebbles can become a castle; a little breeze and a kite have endless possibilities! Our ability, as "grown-ups", to enjoy life is only covered up by the "pressures" (attitudes) of our grown-up life. All we need to do is consciously rediscover the child within us and learn how to play again.

A child lives close to prana, close to inner needs and natural responses that are uncensored by the mind. This same dynamic is experienced as we laugh and play. This is why we, indeed, feel like "kids" when we're experiencing ourselves in this way. Much has been written in the past decade about re-connecting and nurturing "the child

within us" (see appendix). New Age psychology has asserted that we become "adult" too soon and remain in that role too often, mistakenly thinking that our well-being will flourish if we are "mature", if we remain in mental and emotional control. The child, on the other hand, lets go of life. In the act of playing, the body moves naturally and effortlessly; in the act of laughing, the doors of the heart open to joy -- a joy that is inherent in each of us.

We need to rediscover that child within each of us and nurture it, as another step on the path to Holistic Health. The following exercises have been designed to help you do just that.

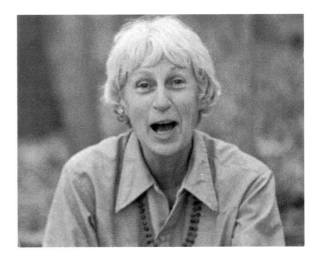

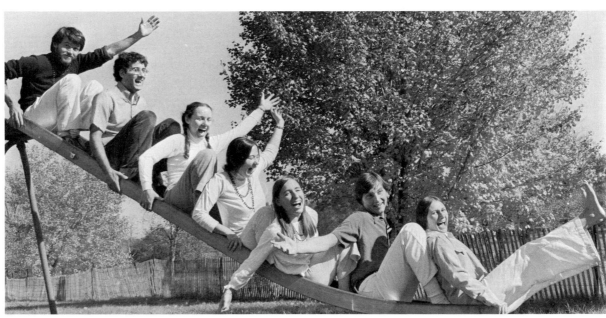

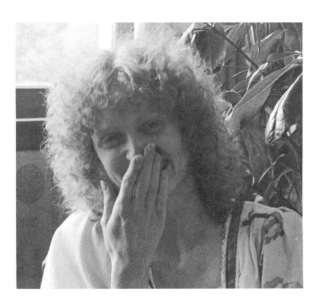
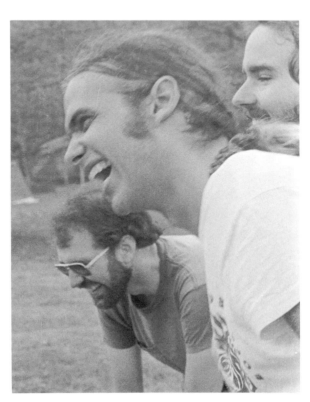
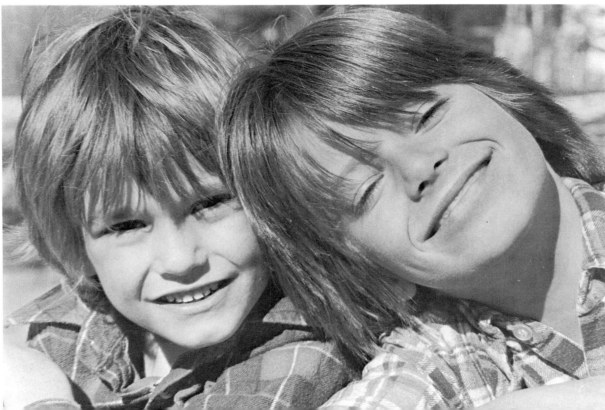

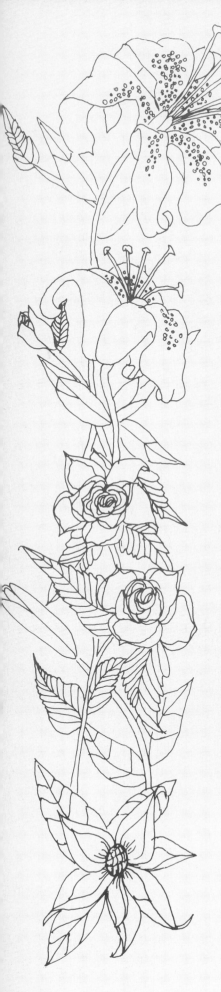

Self–Discovery

Getting To Know the Playful Child Within You

This experience is a little different than previous ones. You will need: 1)Some sheets of sketching paper, 2) lined notebook paper, 3) if possible, some colored crayons or pencils, and 4) a mirror. Be prepared to have some fun!

Awareness

1. First, sit still and see if you can remember something that gave you a real good belly laugh -- perhaps recently, perhaps some time ago. Allow yourself to remember it so vividly (it may help to close your eyes) that you begin to laugh heartily again at the memory. It may take some time, but just relax until you recapture the memory and the feeling. If you are unable to actually re-experience the laughter, then try to recall how your body felt when you laughed. Now, how do you feel, physically, emotionally, mentally? Write it down.

2. If you weren't able to get in touch with your laughter, how does that make you feel right now? How do you respond when other people are laughing and you don't find it funny? Write these thoughts down.

3. Reflect back for a moment. How often do you laugh, really laugh? Is it often enough? Do you sometimes wish you were able to laugh more? Do you wish that more funny/laughable things happened in your life? How do you *feel* about laughter, humor, play and the role they have in your life right now? Write these feelings down also.

4. Now close your eyes after reading these instructions and go through the following visualization. See yourself as a very small child, laughing and playing with other children. Try to feel how it felt to be that child. See how he or she was playing, and feel the emotion and bodily sensations. When you've really immersed yourself in the experience, open your eyes, and *without thinking* start to draw or sketch the images that come to you to express what you experienced in the visualization. It is important to drop any old "tapes" which say, "I can't draw", or "I'm not artistic." Just transfer your images to paper, knowing no one will see them but you. And enjoy it! They may be drawings which depict you as a child, with the toys and games you played; they may be just abstract shapes and images that symbolize the feelings. You can write in single words too, if they seem to fit.

5. Close your eyes again, and repeat the visualization process with a later stage in your childhood -- maybe age 8 or 9. Again, draw the images that come to you spontaneously as you open your eyes, without thinking. Thinking quickly becomes judging and curbs and stifles the innate creativity borne to the surface by prana. Repeat the process three more times, for your teenage years, your young adulthood, and the present moment.

6. Review all your sketches and notes, and see what they spontaneously tell you about yourself, your attitudes to play and humor, and how you have changed over the years. What did you laugh *at,* then and now? How fully did you/do you laugh and how often? Write down your observations.

Experience 10

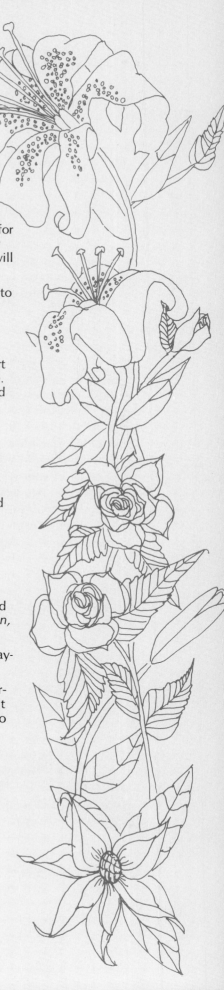

7. Try to see any patterns that are preventing you from being more playful and humorous in the present. Do you have an "inner parent" telling you: "grow up", "be sensible", "stop being childish", "don't be lazy", "don't be silly", "act your age", etc? Do you have old "tapes" in your head which contain the message that playing is just for children, mature adults don't play, or if you want to be respected and taken seriously you can't afford to fool around, to be lighthearted? (These are just suggestions; you will have your own "tapes" which will be different.)

8. Do you really *believe* in play and humor as important parts of life, as contributors to health? Did you in the past?

Acceptance

1. Sitting quietly, just absorb what you have learned about yourself and make it a part of you. Feel good about it, as if that part of you were a new friend you had just made. Feel what it means to you -- how it changes the image you have held of yourself -- and be glad you can now adjust to a more accurate and enjoyable self-concept.

2. Make a drawing of your "inner-child."

3. Speak now to that newly-discovered child who has been hiding inside of you waiting to be allowed out to play. As if you were the loving, nurturing parent of this child, ask him or her:
"What do you need from me? What would you like me to do so that you may express yourself through play and humor?" Then listen to the response of the prana-child and write it down.

4. Now look at yourself in the mirror and smile! Make faces, clown around, be child-like -- and childish. Enjoy your new-found child.

Adjustment

1. Start writing down all the ways in which you can safely express your inner child and meet his/her needs. Be specific, as to *what* you will do, *when, with whom, how often, etc.*

2. Gather ideas from the following "How to" Section to incorporate into your new play-scheme.

3. Resolve to consciously nurture that inner-child, to lovingly support his or her emergence and growth, just as you would have to with a real child -- for it *is* a real child. It is the child that you once were, who had to grow up too soon or who became afraid to express and enjoy itself because the adults around it disapproved of its high spirits (because the child in them had been squashed in their parents and teachers unknowingly). The chain of cause and effect recedes into infinity. Tell your child when you are pleased with him or her and encourage him or her to be daring and fearless, to be real.

10 Ways to Nurture Your Inner Child

1. *Be with children* and play with them or, at least, observe them play. See their total absorption in what they are doing, how "lost" they are in it. See how freely they laugh at the smallest things, not caring what the laughter sounds or looks like. Notice their complete lack of inhibition and self-criticism.

2. *Laugh for the pure pleasure of laughing,* not because something is funny and you are laughing *at* it. You may have to force yourself at first (old habits die hard, they say) and you may feel "phony" or be embarrassed by the sound of your own laughter. In actual fact, your "forced" laughter is more real than your habitual seriousness, for laughter is innate in all of us (and only in humans, perhaps as a gift to counteract our overactive minds). We have simply lost the spontaneity of it. Deep, full laughter involves muscles that haven't been used for a long time and that need practice and remedial exercise!

3. Find yourself a "buddy" to have fun with and practice on each other! Pick someone you trust fully and have no fear of being judged or rejected by, otherwise you won't be able to express yourself fully.

4. *Laugh, don't just smile!* Will Durant said, "The smile is sometimes an abortion of a laugh."

5. *Laugh at yourself.* Cultivate a more detached attitude to your problems and difficulties, so that you can see the humor inherent in almost all situations. Life is not so serious really. Sincerity is one thing, seriousness another.

6. *Look at the world through a child's eyes* -- empty, wondering, marvelling at the ever-new panorama unfolding before you.

7. *Everyday, do something playful,* different, spontaneous. But be careful to choose appropriate people and places. Someone who has not "re-awakened the inner child" may not see the joke.

8. *Read children's books* for their freshness and humor. We especially like *Winnie-the-Pooh* by A.A. Milne, and *The Secret Garden* by Frances Hodgson Burnett. See appendix for other ideas.

9. *Share your joy.* "A sorrow that's shared is but half the trouble, but a joy that's shared is a joy made double."

10. *Play games with yourself and others.* Here's a list to help you get started.

Games to Play Just for the Fun of It

Here are some games we play at the Kripalu Center for Holistic Health, "something old, something new, something borrowed and something blue!"

1. *Card and board games.* Old favorites like Monopoly and Scrabble and New Age games like "Feeling Good."

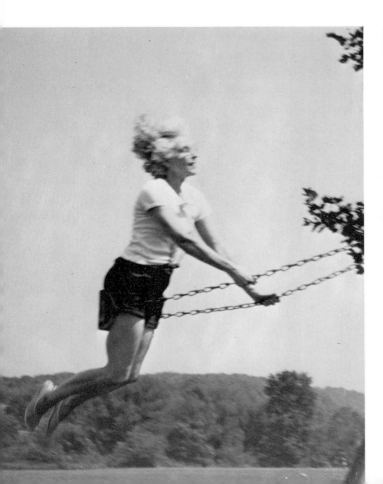

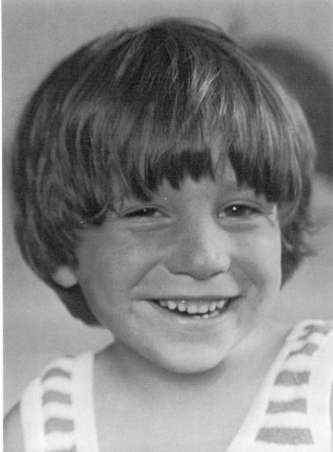

2. Charades (When was the last time *you* played it, and really enjoyed it?)

3. Kids' games like wheelbarrow, sack, and egg and spoon races.

4. Dressup games (remember how you loved to dress up as a kid?)

5. Crazy team games. For example:

(a) Each member has to do something like dress up in old clothes of the opposite sex and race to a point and back.

(b) Each team has 5 minutes to form itself into an animal; then it parades in front of the other team(s) who have to guess its identity.

(c) Two teams face each other. One member from each team must start at each end and as they walk down between the teams, toward the other end and passing each other in the middle, they must not laugh. The rest of the team, of course, is supposed to do everything in its power (short of physical contact) to make their opponents' member laugh or smile. A loser goes to the other team. (Didn't you just *love* this as a kid at a party?)

(d) Tug-of-War.

These are just examples. You can make up your own.

6. "Experience" games. One such game is done in groups of 3 or 4. One person must become totally slack and relaxed; the others are to gently lower that person to the ground, then lift them up to a standing position again. (You won't believe how heavy a totally relaxed body is. Sometimes three other people cannot lift it.) Then have someone tense up their whole body, like a board, and see how easy it is to lift it.

7. Fun by yourself.

(a) When no one's around, put on some dancing music and dance all by yourself. Do it to wear yourself out, to express all your energy, like a high-spirited child.

(b) Run rather than walk sometimes, not like a jogger but like a free child. Skip and jump, jump in puddles, go barefoot, eat with your fingers, sing songs to yourself -- in short, *be a child* for a while.

For more game and book suggestions, see the appendix.

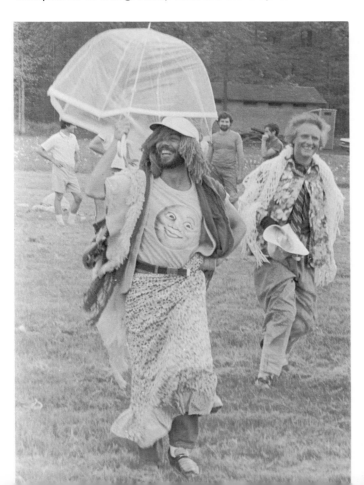

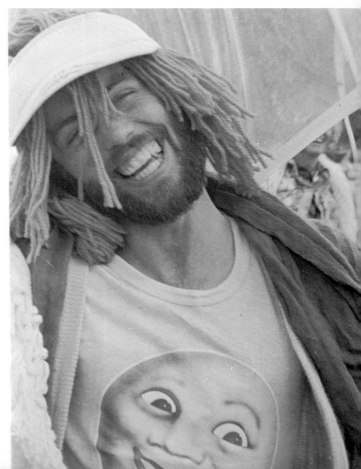

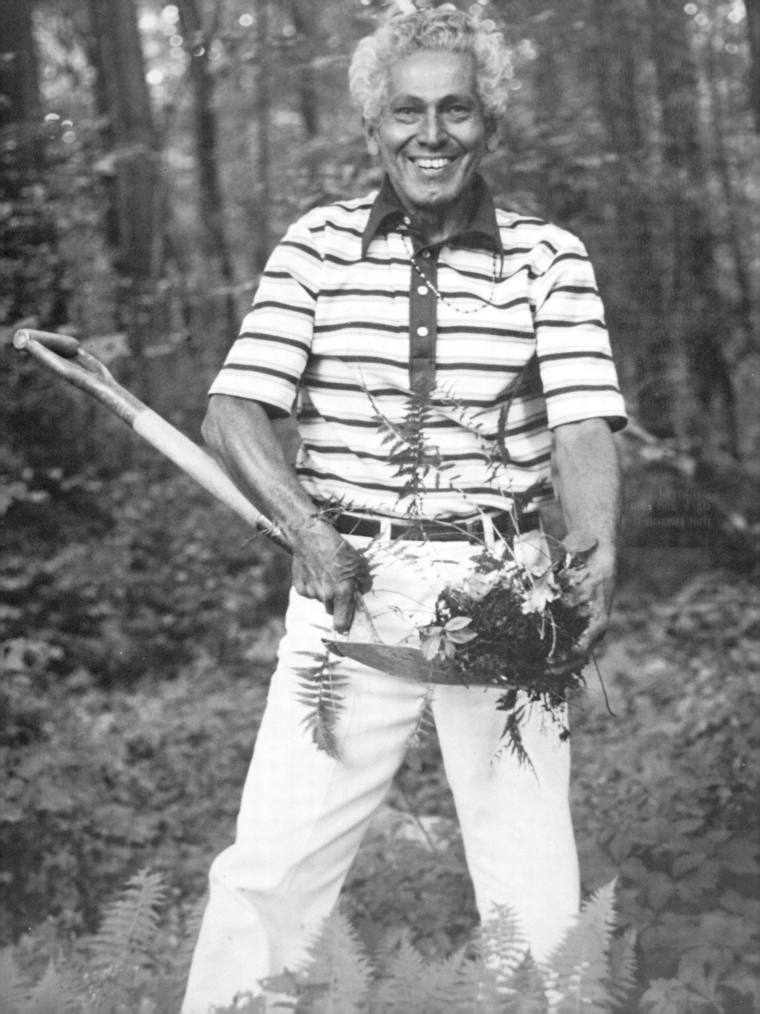

WAY FOUR
the art of relaxed work

WORK: EXPRESSING OUR CREATIVE ENERGY

Eight hours a day, five days a week, fifty weeks a year -- from the time we learn to make our own bed until the time we plant our post-retirement garden -- in all those hours and in all those years, we work; we are doers. Work is an expression of our energy, our body, our mind, our heart, our soul, our creative potential. By its very nature it is holistic. It is no wonder then, that work deserves our attention as a way, a path, to the experience of happiness and well-being in our lives.

The articles and exercises that follow are opportunities for you to explore the place that work holds in your approach to health, and to develop ways to make it contribute more to your well-being and happiness.

Work and Relaxation -- Opposites?

"Work" -- the very word conjures up the opposite of relaxation for many people. However much we may like our jobs, work means effort and relaxation is something that we do on weekends or on vacation (in other words, when we're *not* working). Yet work and relaxation can be blended into a whole. This is a fundamental part of the Kripalu Approach to Holistic Health, the cornerstone of which is free-flowing prana energy. As we have already seen, the key to free-flowing prana is relaxation in everything we do, including (indeed most importantly) work. But how can we be relaxed at work? Some people just are; some jobs seem to preclude it. Loving what you do helps, but even then stress can creep in. Isn't it inevitable that we should feel tired by 5pm every day and exhausted by Friday afternoon? After all, working hard for 40 hours a week or so is tiring isn't it? Not necessarily. Yogi Desai, for instance, puts in more hours a week than almost anyone we know in a normal job. He directs three organizations, counsels and provides spiritual guidance to many, teaches workshops and seminars around the country, yet he *never* seems to be tired. His energy seems to be boundless. What is the secret?

The secret is conservation of energy. That means two things: (1) spending the energy we have cautiously and wisely, not wasting or draining it or letting it leak away unconsciously, and (2) learning to draw in more than the average amount of energy.

There are two main areas to work on in energy conservation. We need to learn to be more consciously aware of what is happening to the energy in our bodies and to examine and change stress-causing attitudes (as we found in the previous chapter). Keeping in touch with the body is explained in more detail in the 7th Way, in an article entitled "The Meditation of Natural Living". In this chapter we will look at the question of what are the attitudes we have about our work which cause us to experience it as tiring and tension producing.

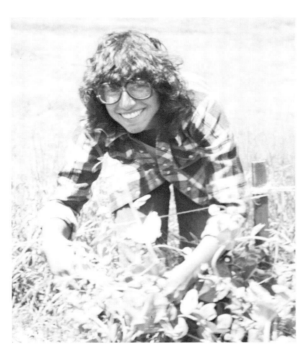

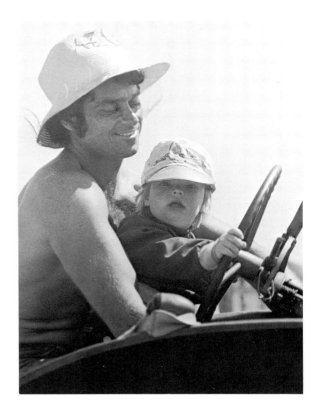

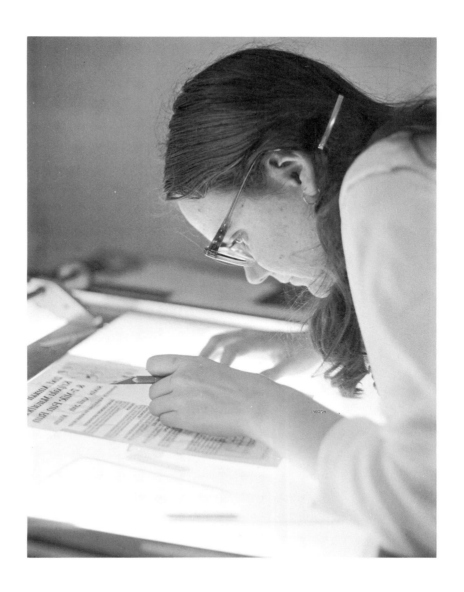

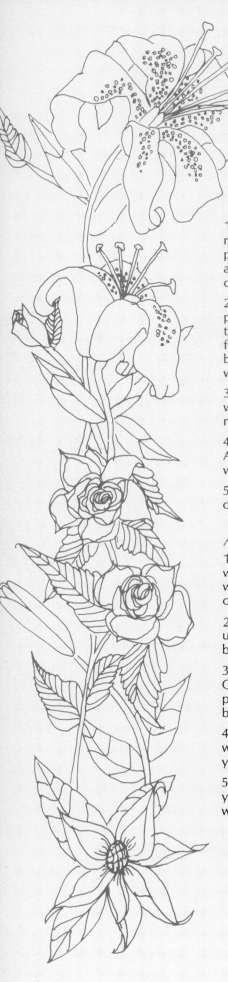

Self-Discovery

What Do Your Hidden Attitudes About Work Reveal To You?

GET PENCIL & PAPER, AND SET ASIDE 30 QUIET MINUTES ALONE TO DO THIS INTROSPECTION.

Awareness

1. Take an inventory of your perceptions and definitions of "work." Close your eyes, relax, and let your mind dwell on what "work" means to you. Then, on a piece of paper, freely list and/or draw the words, phrases and images you associate with the activity called "work." Put down whatever comes, without evaluating, judging or criticizing it.

2. Now see yourself going through a typical work day. Start from the beginning, perhaps as you get out of bed, preparing yourself to go to work. Come in touch with the feelings about "work" that you experience in each phase. List or draw those feelings and the ways they find expression (examples: "frustrated driving to work, so I blew my horn in traffic jam,", "excited about a new project, so I am enthusiastic in talk with Jim," etc.).

3. Now complete the following statement being as honest with yourself as you can: "I work because…" List everything that comes to mind, from the practical reasons to the more subtle.

4. Finally, and honestly, list whom it is important for you to please through your work. After each name, list what it is you hope to receive from this person as a result of your work.

5. If you have more than one kind of "work" (e.g. a housewife who also holds an outside job) explore the differences in attitude you have about your various "jobs".

Acceptance

1. Re-read your response to Section 1 above. For each response, write down what or who it is that has influenced your definitions or perceptions about work. Take stock of which perceptions still appear reasonable when you look at them consciously and objectively.

2. Consider Sections 3, 4 and 5. Look over each list and write down what your true underlying *needs* may be (example: you want your boss to give you a pat on the back, but what you really need is to feel accepted).

3. Consider Sections 4 and 5. Close your eyes and see clearly the persons you listed. Going beyond your formal relationship with them (your role and theirs) be with the person *behind* the title or role. Come in touch with what you sincerely desire to feel between the two of you, and write it down.

4. Consider Section 2 above. Complete the statement: "I express my feelings about my work in this way rather than in another because…" Reflect on how you can increase your awareness of how your feelings influence your behavior and attitudes at work.

5. Re-read all your answers and see to what extent you have a pattern of identifying yourself as what you "do" and basing your self-esteem on that, rather than simply on what you are.

Experience 11

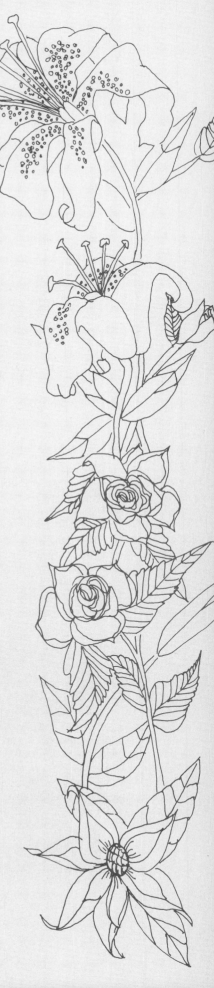

Adjustment

After doing the above exercises you will have a clearer picture of your attitudes and feelings about your work. Re-read all that you have recorded to obtain an overview of who you are as a "doer." Are there any inconsistencies, needs, or perceptions that appear as patterns in each response?

Sitting quietly, let the actions you know you need to take in order to make your work more effective and bring you more happiness emerge from your intuition. Write them down. We all have patterns of response that we could adjust in regard to our work. It is usually best to find the most important one and focus on it first. You may find, for example, a consistent perception that "I should always work hard or others won't value me." Once you have seen this, you can then actually consider whether or not this is true. If you reflect on all your findings in this way, you will discover a whole repertoire of actions you can take to make your work more of a pleasure, and a fuller expression of a wholehearted "you." For example:

1. Re-define what "work" means to you, now. Decide what definition of work you want to live with, one that you think is healthy and reasonable, and let it direct your actions and attitudes as you work.

2. Choose simple, specific ways to reduce tension and conflict. Focus on any pattern of feelings about work that express tension or conflict. Decide on a new way that you can approach this situation. Beginning with the physical is usually the easiest. For example, choose to do deep breathing during the traffic jam. After relaxing, you may get in touch with the real reason for your tension. If it's because you need to talk with your boss about giving you fifteen minutes leeway in arriving in the morning, you're now calm and trusting enough to do so.

3. Choose some ways to share your needs and fears with others. After being clear about what it really is you would like to receive from the significant people in your life, consider ways to share your true needs with them. Your own deeply felt honesty may result in them being able to be more open with you. You will then know what their needs are and how they can be met through a more open communication or relationship.

4. See clearly how you can change your own attitudes. Last, but not least, you may discover that the simplest and yet most powerful way to change your experience of work is to change the way you perceive it.

FREEING YOURSELF FROM "WORK"

Looking at Your Expectations

In the final analysis, it is the concepts that we have about "work", the attitudes with which we approach it, that decree how much satisfaction, pleasure and fulfillment we get. In addition to physical relaxation, we need to cultivate an *attitude* of relaxation toward our work. This does not mean becoming passive and never trying to get ahead, to improve efficiency, or to make a career. It means checking out our underlying attitudes ongoingly, seeing where these cause us to experience tension, and relaxing them.

The most common tension-producing attitude, yet perhaps the one we are least aware of, is expectation. Without realizing it, we expect to get our work done in a certain amount of time, with the complete cooperation of other people and external circumstances. If we are another kind, we expect nothing to go wrong. We expect praise or we expect blame; we expect a promotion or a criticism. Whatever it is, good or bad, we are always expecting, unconsciously. This creates permanent tension in us. Will we or won't we get "it"? How can we avoid "it"? So the first step in learning to enjoy our work more is to drop, or at least become very aware of, our expectations and to simply become absorbed in the moment-to-moment completion of each task in the best possible way.

Focusing on the Process Rather Than the Results

The second most common cause of tension, very probably, is being result-oriented. Of course, we have to care about the results of our labor and to put forth our best effort -- nothing less is worthy of us as conscious beings. Yet we often tend to focus so much of our energy and attention on the final result, that we do not, and cannot, enjoy the process. If we think all the time of how nice "it" will be when "it" is finished, or are anxious about the result, we take ourselves out of the present and lose the pleasure of the moment. Relaxation can only truly come when we are in the *experience of the moment,* not the *thought of the future.* We tend, in the West, to be excessively time-conscious. If we observe ourselves minutely as we go about our daily tasks, we will catch ourselves with many thoughts of "how quickly can I get this task done and move on." We constantly time-pressure ourselves, yet imagine it is the job, the boss, the client, the family, that demand too much of us.

Re-aligning Your Values

This time-consciousness is closely related to, or based upon, a value-consciousness which is also tension-producing. "This task is more important/interesting/valuable/worth my time than that one." "This job is not as rewarding as his/hers." "If only I had a more fulfilling job, I'd be happy." Undeniably, some jobs are more intrinsically interesting than others. Yet our attitude is more important. Without the right attitude, no job, however fascinating, will ever satisfy us because every job has its other side (the chores, the repetition, or perhaps the dangers and tensions).

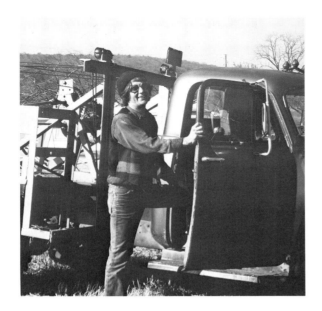

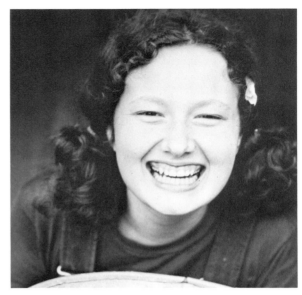

This inappropriate value system comes from identifying ourselves too closely with what we do. "Who are you?" "I am an executive." "I am a housewife." "I am a student." We need to remember we are not what we do. What we do is simply an expression of our energy -- one of many. Of course, this pattern started very early in life. Even in grade school, we felt good about ourselves if we got an 'A', and bad if we got a 'C or 'D'. Our need to do, to succeed, to accomplish, is often simply an expression of our deep human need to feel accepted. Unfortunately, if we work with an unconscious motivation of gaining love and acceptance we will always experience the tension generated by an underlying fear of not getting that acceptance.

There is one source of tension which is perhaps the most potent and yet the hardest for us to see objectively. It runs like a thread through all the other sources. This tension comes from our only being able to see work as a transaction in which we must come out ahead. Unconsciously we are always asking, "What am I getting out of it? Am I being paid enough? Am I getting the respect/gratitude which I deserve?" This is a mistaken viewpoint because it generates tension. Actually, we can seldom be sure that we are getting what is "due" to us. At moments of success, such as receiving a promotion, pay increase, or special praise, it may feel that way, but these are infrequent. So tension will underly our work whenever we are looking at it only in terms of our own gain. If we can, instead, focus on ways in which our work is a service to others, is a giving rather than a getting, we will automatically become more relaxed.

GUIDELINES FOR A MORE RELAXED WORKING LIFE

1. Remain physically relaxed by stopping to do stretching or deep breathing through the day. Get plenty of exercise and fresh air. Make every movement of your body flowing and harmonious, conserving as much energy as possible.

2. Observe your tensions, and use them as messages from which you can learn about yourself.

3. Become conscious of your expectations. If you see them clearly, they won't prevent you from fully accepting and enjoying what is actually happening.

4. Focus more on the moment-to-moment process of what you are doing and less on the end result, which will take care of itself if you are fully efficient in each moment.

5. Let time be your friend, not a constant opponent with which you are fighting. Get lost in the moment, lift the pressure of self-imposed deadlines, plan realistically, and do your best -- in each moment. Then, drop any anxiety. What more can you do than your best?

6. Concentrate on drawing your self esteem, your sense of identity *from all that you are* as a unique individual on this earth, rather than from what you do. See what you do as simply a partial expression of your energy.

7. See all tasks as of equal value in terms of your growth as a whole person. How well you do something, and with what care and attention, is of more importance and value than the mere label attached to the task. Of course this won't come at once, but you can practice.

8. Begin to look at your work in terms of how it can help others. Imagine, as you do something routine, the satisfaction and pleasure someone will ultimately receive from your wholehearted, giving action. For instance, if you are folding laundry, really feel how much pleasure the person will receive as they see and smell the neatly-folded laundry. Or if you're writing a memo, imagine how well-informed and helped the recipient is going to feel, even if you never hear it from them.

See your work as service, in the highest sense of the word, to others and to yourself. By helping others to the best of your ability, with a loving and open heart, you are helping yourself to grow into a happier, more relaxed, more free and fully alive human being. This is what we all want, deep down.

The cumulative effect of making all these small changes of attitude towards your work will be very powerful. You will begin, quite rapidly, to find yourself being more relaxed and able to flow through the day without getting ruffled by things that would formerly have bothered you. You will be less tired and tense by the end of the day, and have more energy to do the other things for which you've always wanted to find time. You will feel in tune with your prana, relaxed and flowing. You will be learning to be more and more in the moment, so that time passes unnoticed and boredom and tension become things of the past.

APPLYING THE PRINCIPLES OF KARMA YOGA TO YOUR WORK

by Yogi Amrit Desai

Karma Yoga is an attitude rather than an action. It is an important attitude, to work and to life, which is well worth cultivating if we wish to achieve Holistic Health, because it will enable us to experience complete freedom from tension. This is the state in which our prana flows freely and our mind, body and spirit are functioning in perfect harmony.

Dropping Anxiety About Results

What is this attitude? How is it different from the way we normally perform our work? Karma Yoga is carrying out our daily tasks and responsibilities, whether at home or at work, in a spirit of equanimity, without entertaining in our mind any anxiety about the results of our actions. It means cultivating a calm and accepting attitude, no matter what happens. It means being dispassionate about the end result (whether fear of failure, desire for success, or simply wanting things to happen in the way that we choose.) If we worry about the results, then our passions and our emotions are constantly involved in what is happening. As a result, we are always carrying tension within us.

Modern Westerners have become very result-oriented. That is why the level of tension in this society is so high. So many people base their whole lives on achieving "success", on meeting specific goals within a specific time frame. It is not wrong to have a sense of direction and commitment. On the contrary, these are very important aspects of life. But there is a big difference between a goal and a direction; between commitment and attachment. Goals and attachments bring us tension and suffering; direction and commitment bring self-knowledge and inner peace.

Seeing Work as Service

To many people, it seems impossible, given the conditions of their lives and occupations in our tense society, to attain to this ideal level of equanimity and calm acceptance of whatever happens. Yet it is really not so difficult once we understand the concept of Karma Yoga. It only takes time, practice and patience. A new attitude needs to be developed: one of selfless service. This means looking at our activities at work in terms of how they can be of help to others, rather than how they can further our own success and reputation. When we are able to drop our own egotistical motives, we immediately dissolve all our work

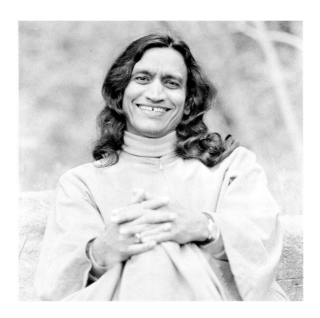

tensions because we no longer have any anxiety about results. Then we can work with relaxation and equanimity, gaining our satisfaction from helping others.

Our life was given to us to help others, not simply to help ourselves. Giving and receiving is a law of nature, and whenever we experience unhappiness in life it is because we have gone against that law and tried to receive more than we gave. Unhappiness is nature's way of reminding us that we must participate in the universal law of giving and receiving. Deep in our hearts, we know this. We feel good about ourselves when we give to others and help them, and we feel bad about ourselves when we ignore the needs of others and step over them to achieve our own ends. Most of our unhappiness and self-rejection comes from a deep inner awareness that we do not consciously recognize. We are subtly aware that we are always wanting something for ourselves and are seldom able to perform any action that is truly selfless.

Dropping the Achievement Syndrome

Everyone wants to be happy. We believe that what will make us happy is the approval, acceptance and love of others. We also believe that to get that approval and acceptance, we must be successful and achieve things. So we spend our lives striving to achieve more and more. We look for success, influence, money, position, hoping that when we achieve these things, we will feel "happy", we will feel accepted and loved by others. We do not see how many people we ignore and reject in our desire to achieve our goals. These goals are not just those of business and career; they are also the goals of society, such

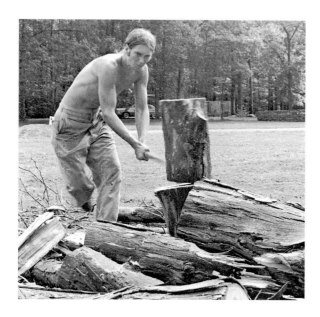

more than anxiety about the results. It also removes anxiety about whether we will receive enough for our services. We know from the start that material reward is not the main purpose; the main purpose is to help others and that satisfaction is received at every moment, as we perform each action.

When we begin to give more of ourselves to others, through our work, we begin to experience a deep sense of satisfaction and fulfillment. Not only do we feel more acceptance from others because we don't want anything from them, but we also begin to accept ourselves, because we know, deep down, we are responding to our true inner nature, to our inborn desire to give to others. This is why wise men have always said that it is in giving that we receive. We receive the benefits of following our own pure, inner nature.

In selfless service we escape from the circle, from the constant need to achieve and get credit for our actions in order to feel accepted. We no longer have to depend on someone else to accept and approve of us before we can accept and approve of ourselves. Of course it will not happen at once just because we have read and understood an article like this. For a while we may still find ourselves looking to others for approval -- this time of our selflessness! But gradually, as we practice making our work a service, we will move out of that stage into an ever greater feeling of freedom and joy.

as to have good relationships, happy marriages, children to be proud of, a nice home, etc. So, we ignore the many whose opinion we consider unimportant, on the outside chance of being accepted by the few whose approval we value.

It's a poor exchange. Not only that, it doesn't work. Even when we achieve the goals we have set our hearts on, we don't experience the satisfaction and fulfillment that we imagined we would -- or not for long. At first, we may feel accepted, even loved, by those around us. Then we begin to see, little by little, that often other people are making us feel good because they want something from us. The acceptance they show is not real -- it is not for us, as people. It is for what we have achieved, and what we possess. Many successful people ultimately, at the end of their lives, find that success is an illusion. It has not brought them happiness.

Substituting Self-Acceptance for Approval

Not only that, even if we do experience true acceptance from others, it will still be no substitute for our own self-acceptance. We will still feel unsatisfied, unfulfilled at a deeper level. We may feel that we are still not as successful as someone else, or not as successful as we want to be. Until we learn to accept ourselves fully no amount of external acceptance, approval and love will make us truly happy. We are unable even to see that we don't accept ourselves. One way to learn to accept ourselves is through selfless service, Karma Yoga. Paradoxically enough, when we completely forget our own needs and serve others, we have a greater ability to accept ourselves, to feel fulfilled and content with who we are and what we are doing with our lives. Selfless service removes

Selfless Service -- The Key to Lasting Happiness

Sometimes it may be hard to see our work as service to others. We may feel we don't have that kind of job, but all actions are service if they are inspiring to others. If we perform all our actions with total commitment, pouring in all our energies, physical, mental and emotional, and doing it with a joyful heart, we will truly be serving others, because they will feel our energy and be inspired by it. When we do something with enthusiasm, sincerity and detachment from the results, we ignite a flame of inspiration among those around us, and they will love us for it.

This attitude of energetic commitment is what distinguishes the acceptance of Karma Yoga from mere passivity. Karma Yoga says that we are to do everything that we can, with total dedication and creativity, yet without feeling any anxiety about the results. This enthusiastic and energetic detachment is the key to true success in life -- the success of lasting inner happiness, independent of all external events. This is the secret of Karma Yoga.

TRANSFORMING WORK INTO SERVICE

By Yogi Amrit Desai

In life we constantly strive for understanding, acceptance and love from others. Yet often we find ourselves frustrated in our efforts. The more we fail to get what we need, the harder we try, until we create such a strong need to receive that we forget to give. Yet this constant desire to receive is the greatest obstacle to receiving what we need. When we are selfish we suffer the consequences of violating one of nature's most basic laws, the law of giving and receiving.

Giving: The First Law of Nature

In the world of nature there is continuous exchange, a never-ending pattern of giving and receiving in which everything changes constantly and nothing remains stagnant. The ocean receives water from the sky only to give off water, which is then drawn up into the sky again. The water, transformed into rain, is given to the rivers and eventually returns to the ocean. The trees give their seeds to the earth, which nourishes and sustains the seeds and eventually gives forth new trees. This continuous pattern of giving and receiving has only one exception: human beings, who alone violate this law and replace it with the unnatural laws of the individual ego. When we violate nature's laws by receiving more than we give, the lost harmony of nature within us sends signals that an imbalance has been created. These signals come to us as feelings of fear, loneliness, frustration, or depression. Through each of these experiences, nature is trying to direct our attention to the basic disharmony we have created in and around ourselves, through our unconscious selfishness.

Taking -- The First Law of Ego

Selfishness is the first law of the ego, and the source of much of the conflict, separateness and loneliness that we experience. When selfishness burns, the light of love dissolves into the darkness of ignorance. No other form of ignorance can hurt as deeply as selfishness.

Selfishness says: "I want you to understand me, whether I understand you or not. I want you to accept me, whether I accept you or not. I want you to love me, whether I love you or not." Selfishness knows only one way: the way of receiving. It makes us blind to the needs of others. We see only ourselves; others are only means to fulfill our own personal dreams.

The stronger our desire for what we want, the more we forget to give to others. This selfishness may even drive us to ignore, use and ultimately hurt others in an attempt to fulfill our own cherished dreams. Yet these dreams and desires can never be fully satisfied; we will never get "enough". Once we become gripped in the jaws of our own selfish desires, we ceaselessly strive for more, continuously working, in fear, to protect what we have already achieved. In such striving there is no arriving -- no point of satisfaction and satiation. Our consciousness has become caught in the vicious cycle of endless striving, and endless wanting.

Trapped in the Web of Self-Interest

We do not do this intentionally, for we do not want to ignore or hurt others. Yet, as soon as we experience a powerful desire for something, be it an external possession or position, or a specific response from another, we automatically view others according to their ability to provide what we want. Ironically, we are often the last to realize what we are doing. We play games without knowing that we play games. Others may recognize our games, but we ourselves are unable to see them. So we become more deeply trapped in our own web of dishonesty and self-interest. We find ourselves in greater and greater conflict with others, yet we are unable to recognize the source of the conflict as being within ourselves. Such is the blindness of selfishness.

Selfishness and loneliness are synonymous. When we are selfish, we feel alone and are separate from others. In order to feel the closeness that we need, we seek others' understanding of us; we try to win the understanding or acceptance of the other rather than to give to the other. Yet, we also unconsciously realize that we will only get what we want from the other by appearing to be

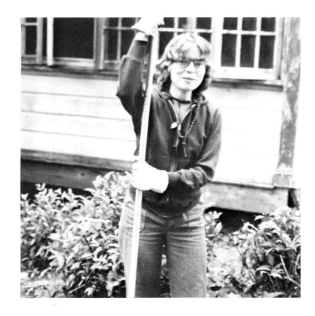

selfless in every possible way. We know that the other will accept and trust us to the degree that we appear to be selfless, and so we put on the garb of selflessness.

Our Secret Lists of Wants

When people first meet, they are usually wearing the garb of selflessness. Each gives to the other, thinking of what the other wants and striving to meet the needs of the other. But each person has two secret lists: a list of their own needs and a list of what they believe to be the other's needs. If they think they will get what they want from the other, they act as though they can give the other what he or she wants. They don't put their own list first, but secretly they watch how the needs on their own list are being met. Neither one is seeing the true characteristics of the other person. Each is seeing only the facade that the other has adopted in order to make sure that his or her own needs are met. This facade has been designed unconsciously and the real person hidden unintentionally, but eventually it becomes a habitual way of behaving. When people are new to each other they generally allow their own selfish needs to recede into the background. But habits are habits, and they cannot be hidden for long without a lot of strain and effort. So eventually people begin to let their own selfish needs come to the front again and conflict develops. This dynamic happens as much in work relationships as in personal relationships. Everyone is constantly trying to experience the joy of closeness with others and, at the same time, they are trying to keep their distance so that they can protect their own selfish dreams. Each person fears that if they let others come too close they will not be accepted as they really are. So we cannot live with each other, and yet we cannot live without each other either. We cannot tolerate closeness, yet we cannot bear the pain of feeling separate from others either. We live in constant inner conflict.

The Solution: Selfless Service

The solution is to learn to reduce our selfish desires, and learn true selflessness, rather than putting on the appearance of selflessness. If you learn to give, your receiving is already hidden in it. Such giving is an art. Only when you learn to give without expectations of return does your giving become instant receiving. The receiving begins before you even start to give because this kind of receiving is happening inside you. You experience the rehearsal of giving as you imagine how your giving will help, and your inner joy brings such a transformation in you that you begin to receive automatically and spontaneously before you even give. Such a deep joy in giving is the purest gift, one that very few are able to experience. The true art of receiving what you really want is the art of giving. Here are six ways in which you can learn to be more selfless.

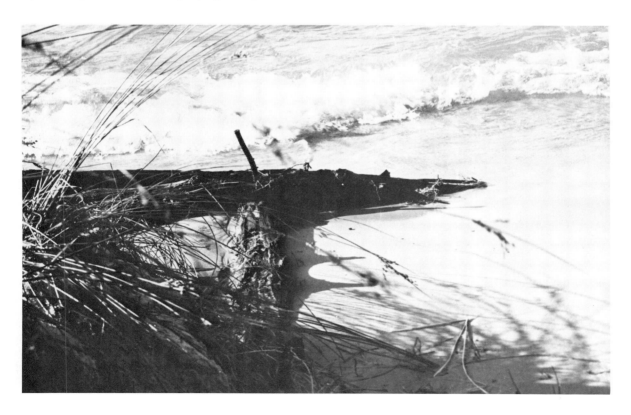

SIX STEPS TO SELFLESS SERVICE

1. Recognize Others' Needs

Learning to be selfless is a lifelong practice. In the beginning you do not need to let go of all your wants; you simply need to recognize the needs of the other also. The first stage of learning selflessness is the willingness to have a fair exchange. At this stage you have a combination of selfishness and selflessness. You are selfish to a degree -- you want something for yourself -- but you also wish to give. And you begin to see the other in terms of what he needs, with compassion.

2. First, Accept Others' Selfishness

Your own selfishness will not be understood or accepted by others unless you are willing to understand and accept their selfishness. But if both say, "I want to be understood first" there is no meeting ground for either one. Only by being first willing to accept the other's selfishness can you initiate the process by which the other can also accept it and become free of it, not by satisfying it but by understanding it.

Love and selfishness are diametrical opposites, yet most people make constant efforts to mix both in every relationship. You want to get something out of that relationship and you also want it to be a loving relationship. It never happens, because selfishness is the invisible wall that separates you from love. The dawn of love is the death of selfishness.

3. Constantly Give Out the Love You Receive

You cannot receive unless you give. If you receive love and acceptance, you must constantly give it out in return. In the process of giving and receiving you are continuously being emotionally flushed out and all your impurities are washed away. But if you only receive you become clogged and unable to receive further. If you fill your pail with water and neglect to empty it, the water will become stagnant and the pail will be unable to take in new, fresh water. In the same way, the container of love that is your heart cannot cling to the love it receives without becoming stagnant. You must be ready to give the love you receive. Be a channel, not a container.

4. Give More Than You Think You Are Receiving

Selfishness is the source of many conflicts and misunderstandings. The whole purpose of personal or spiritual growth is to learn to let go of this selfishness and gradually become able to give. As you progress in this learning process you must go past the stage of fair exchange and gradually become willing to have an *unfair* exchange. That willingness must exist for a relationship to work, because as long as both people expect a fair exchange each one remains focused on the unfairness of the other. One person must be willing to have a bad deal if love is to last. You must be willing to be cheated, consciously knowing what you are doing, realizing what is happening as you let go. Then your losing becomes winning, because now your entire value system is different.

5. Serve Without Seeking Any Return

For you, the benefit is not in getting what you want, but in learning to consciously let go of your selfishness. As you experience this letting go, you begin to see that receiving happens for you in a very strange way. Externally you may not receive anything, yet internally you begin to receive the essence of all you really want, which is peace, comfort, fulfillment. Externally you may have even lost a great deal, but internally you receive the results of success as you experience satisfaction, contentment and joy.

Service is a very direct and simple way to learn selflessness. The basic idea behind service is that you give without asking for a return. Such service is the antidote to conflict, the antidote to separateness, loneliness, and fear of the other.

Service is an unfailing tool which invariably shows you where you are being egotistical and where you are not truly giving. Most conflicts you come across as you serve are the direct outcome of your own selfishness. If in the past you have been excessively selfish, you will encounter more conflicts in service. Those are not new conflicts. You are simply beginning to see the conflicts and selfishness already buried inside you, and service is the mirror which allows you to see. The purpose of seeing your selfishness is to enable you to gradually become free through understanding.

6. Serve in Areas In Which You Seek Growth

In deciding where you will offer your service there is one basic principle to follow: choose the source from which you wish to receive. Once you begin to give your service you will invariably begin to receive from that source also, because it is impossible to separate giving and receiving. If you give service or even financial support to an organization you become subtly connected to that organization and the effects of its work return to you in a variety of ways. You become part of whomever you serve.

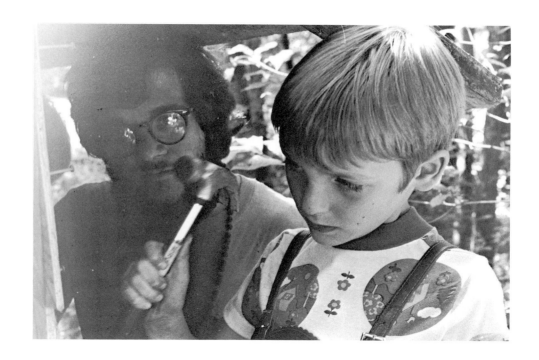

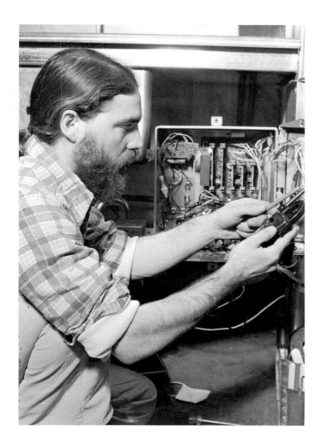

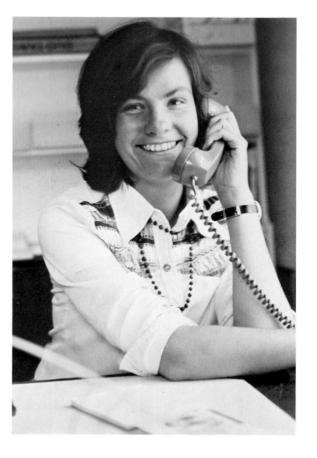

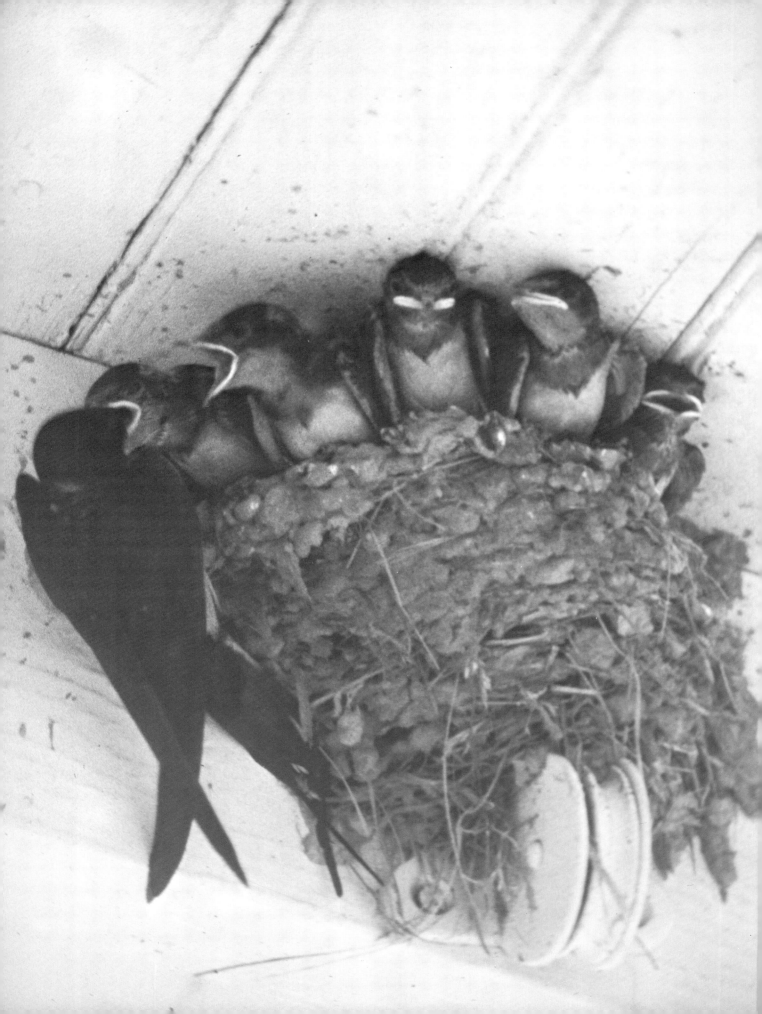

WAY FIVE

discovering your own optimum diet

EATING RIGHT AND EATING WELL -- YOUR OWN WAY

There are, by now, so many books and magazines about diet and nutrition on the market that one of them has been aptly entitled *Are You Confused?* And certainly many people are confused. These books have been written, for the most part, by sincerely motivated people, many of whom are experts. Their theories are based on scientific findings and sound experimentation, yet they seem to disagree on all but the most fundamental facts. So who are we to believe? Why is there so much disagreement? How are we to know what is really the best, most nutritious diet for us? How can we learn to discriminate between the many different options available to us? How can we find our own optimum diet?

This chapter addresses itself to these questions. Rather than add to your confusion (if indeed you are confused; you may be one of the lucky ones who are not) it will help you to resolve it. The Kripalu Approach does not come out in favor of any one diet over any other, for all have their merits. Instead, it teaches a new approach to nutrition which will enable you to become free of diets and nutrition plans devised by other people, even if they are experts, forever. It will give you the liberating experience of becoming your own nutritional expert by learning to hear the messages of your own personal, inner diet doctor, your prana.

The emphasis, as always in this book, is on you and your personal experience. With this in mind, start off by completing the Self-Discovery Experience which follows. It may lead you into a totally new perspective on eating.

After that, you will find we have separated the discussion on nutrition into two distinct areas. The first is the conventional one. It focuses on *what* you eat and reviews the kinds of foods that are beneficial (and not so beneficial) to health. The second area of discussion is special to the Kripalu Approach. It focuses on *how* and *why* you eat. This is a key area that is missing from so many otherwise good approaches to diet and nutrition.

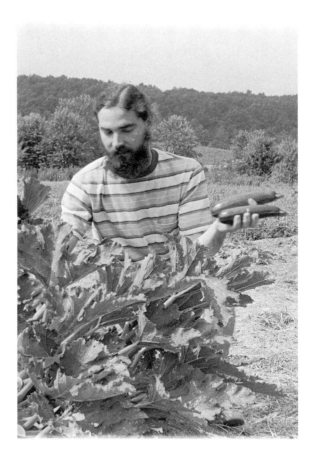

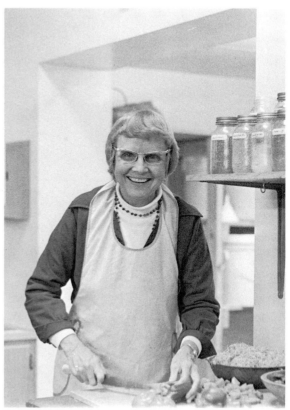

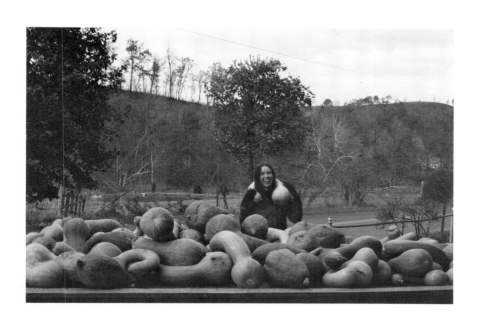

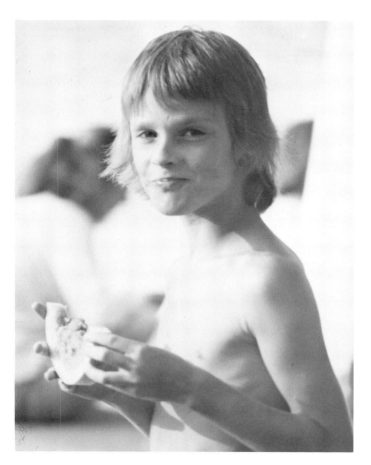

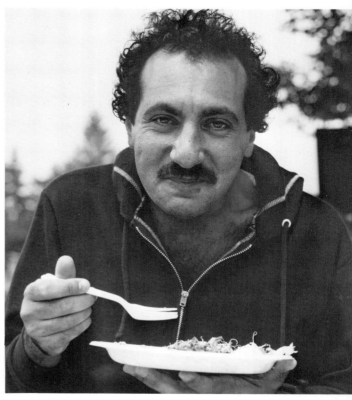

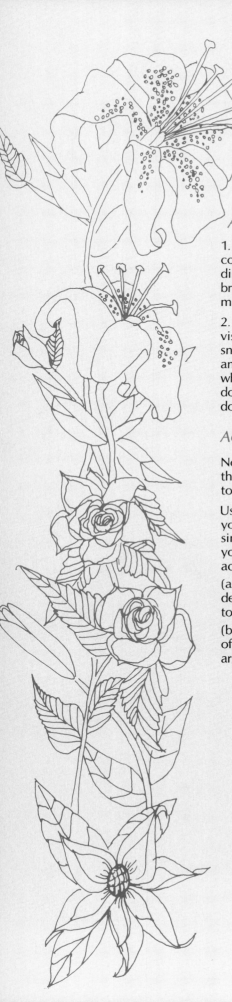

Self–Discovery

What Can You Learn From Your Eating Patterns?

Awareness

1. Sitting quietly, with your eyes closed, begin to let thoughts and associations connected with "food" and "eating" flow through your mind, without judging them or directing them. Simply let them happen to you. Write them down as they come, in brief catch phrases, or draw them. Then close your eyes again. Do this for about 5 minutes.

2. Now, again in your mind's eye, see yourself going through a typical day and visualize all the times that you stopped to take any form of food or drink, be it meal or snack. Each time, consciously recall how you were feeling, what you were thinking and doing before, during and after the meal, snack, or drink. Notice particularly whether you were calm and relaxed, tense, tired, emotional, hungry, bored, etc. Write down or draw each of these "food events" as you recall them (e.g. "at 11am ate a doughnut and drank coffee -- needed a break from work").

Acceptance

Now re-read, item by item, what you have written thus far, objectively noting anything that you observe, recognize or learn from what you see. Just write down what comes to mind, without puzzling over it too much or criticizing it.

Using the questions below as a guideline, try to see the habit patterns that govern your eating. Be really honest, but do not judge what you see as "good" or "bad" -- simply see it clearly for what it is. (If you tend to feel guilty easily, you won't allow yourself to see clearly so as to avoid these unpleasant guilt feelings. If you can just accept without judging, then everything will be crystal clear.)

(a) How often do I eat from real hunger, real physical need, and how often from habit, desire, need for pleasurable taste sensations, to combat boredom, to console myself, to take away or dissipate negative emotions such as fear, anger, depression, etc.?

(b) How often do I eat slowly, peacefully, and quietly, in relaxed surroundings? How often do I eat "on the run", hurriedly, with tension or anger, while discussing or arguing, while reading or watching TV, while listening to the radio, etc.?

Experience 12

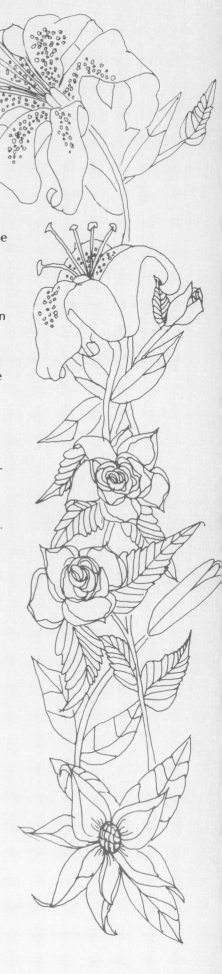

(c) How often do I *really* taste and enjoy every morsel, and how often do I find I've eaten a whole meal almost without noticing?

(d) How often do I stop when I know I've had enough and how often do I go on because it tastes so good, because I don't want to go back to what I need to do after eating, or because I have nothing else to do?

(e) How often do I feel alert and pleasantly satisfied after a meal and how often do I feel uncomfortably full, have indigestion, or feel sleepy and dull?

(f) How often do I eat healthy, nutritious, "live" foods and how often do I "junk out" on artificial, processed, sweet, carbohydrate-heavy, or nutritionless foods?

Go over all that you have written so far and try to observe some typical patterns in your eating. Are there specific times of day, days of the week, or situations where you can observe yourself eating less well than at other times? Note these patterns and write them down.

Adjustment

Read the sections on "How to Practice Conscious Eating" and choose some ways in which you can begin to change your eating habits so that they are more conducive to your health and well-being. Bite off only what you can chew! Just start in small ways -- perhaps relaxing for a few minutes before each meal, cutting back on the amount of coffee that you drink, or deciding to snack less between meals. Just *be aware*. Begin to constantly watch how and when you eat and what you eat, and see what more you can learn from it. Most of all, drop any guilt feelings that come from eating "wrongly". It's better to eat the "wrong" thing, with relaxation and enjoyment, than to feel guilty and self-rejecting about it. Perhaps it is even better than eating the right thing with resentment, longing and tension. Feel good about yourself. After all, who said you had to be perfect?

WHAT YOU EAT -- YOUR FOOD

You Are Unique

Many of life's experiences slip by us without teaching us anything because we are not alert enough to be objectively aware of what is happening to us as it is happening. We are then unable to integrate these experiences at a deeper level, where they can affect our total being and enable us to make the necessary adaptive changes that will improve the quality of our lives.

Among the many diet and nutrition books on the market, there is none superior to our own body when it comes to finding our own, personal, optimum diet for physical, mental and spiritual well-being. The wide range of books and diet programs available often ends up creating further confusion, simply because we don't know whom to believe or where to begin. Each expert disagrees with the next on all but the most fundamental points. There are three main reasons for this. First, they were all writing for different people and cultures, at different times and places. Second, no matter how well-schooled the expert is, he or she is still interpreting the facts through a set of personal, subjective, experiential filters. And third, everyone is different -- a book or a diet has, of necessity, been developed for many people based on the "average" person. The average person does not exist. Everyone's requirements are different. Each person's history, metabolism, and energy needs are unique.

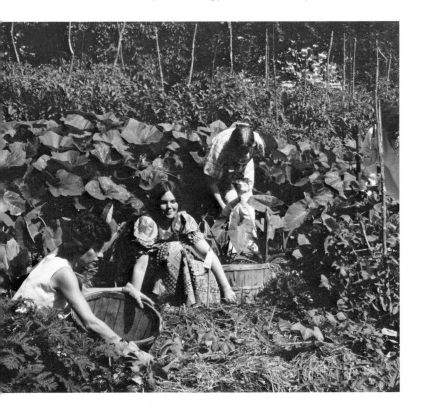

Prana: Your Own Inner Nutrition Specialist

Clearly, the ultimate answer is to learn to rely on our own inner body wisdom, our prana, for guidance. Unfortunately, as we have seen, most of us have forgotten how to read the signals of prana. Its language is a lost art. We don't even hear it until it shouts at us through the unmistakable language of pain, and then our first response is frequently to try and "shut the pain up" by taking remedies -- antacids, painkillers, whatever -- rather than to see the pain as a messenger and learn to understand what it is telling us. This is where the Kripalu Approach differs from most others. Rather than prescribing another set of food rules, it teaches us two things: 1) how to tune in to that personal, inner nutrition specialist called prana, and 2) how to interpret what prana teaches.

How can you re-learn this lost ability to communicate with your prana about the food your body needs? It can be accomplished by informed and guided personal experimentation. There are two distinct stages in this process of arriving at a personal diet which is optimally supportive of Holistic Health. The first stage is transitional. While learning to develop an informed sensitivity to your body's needs, it is still necessary to follow a set of externally-proposed guidelines for appropriate nutrition, but always with flexibility and heightened awareness. At this stage, your own perceived signals will often be misleading. They may be caused by habitual desires and preferences rather than by genuine bodily needs. You may crave something sweet, for instance, when your body really needs protein. You graduate to the second stage when you have learned to interpret the language of your body really well. Then you can confidently listen to your own prana, your own inner intuition of needs, and develop the diet that is uniquely suited to you and no one else.

Your Food Is Your Medicine

Many ancient peoples knew that food is medicine -- not just because herbs can be used to cure various ills, but because the proper diet helps to keep the body in a constant state of optimal health. Ancient India's Ayurvedic system of medicine was based on this belief, and yoga has always taught that our level of consciousness is determined in part by what we put into our bodies. Modern science has discovered that every single cell in the human body is replaced over a period of 7 years and that these new cells are made up of the nourishment that we have taken into our bodies. So we are, literally, what we eat.

To understand how your food affects your consciousness, you need first to learn what happens to the food that you take into your body. There are three possibilities. Some food is digested and then turned into either fuel for the body or new tissue. Some is excreted. Some is retained in the body, yet is useless. It may become fatty deposits, which are usually highly visible, but it may also linger as toxic material lodged invisibly in or around the cells of the body, sapping vitality, fogging the mind and emotions, and causing disease and premature aging.

Prana and Purification

There are two ways to eliminate these toxins from the body: 1) purifying your diet so that you only take in what you need and can use or excrete, and 2) purifying your body of accumulated toxins and waste products. Purifying the diet must be done gradually, so as not to shock your system too much, for the body is a creature of habit and likes its familiar foods. It is necessary, for this purification process, to know two things: (a) which foods are generally agreed, by most sources, to be harmful and (b) the general effect on the body-mind of different categories of food. In the first category, that of harmful foods, come additives of all kinds, refined products such as white flour and white sugar and red meats (some, of course, say all animal flesh, as is our belief, however a transition diet can include moderate amounts of poultry and fish). Meat is better avoided because it often contains harmful substances, such as hormones fed to fatten the animals and adrenalin released by their fear at the moment of death. Both are unhealthy for humans. There are many stages to dietary purification; many vegetarians come to a stage where they wish to eliminate all dairy products too, but this is an optional later stage.

Diet and Energy

It is also useful to know that certain types of food provide specific types of energy to your body. A little self-observation will illustrate this. Rich, heavy foods (such as many pasta dishes, steaks with rich sauces, breads, and pastries and cakes) will tend to leave you feeling rather heavy and lethargic, as will alcohol, when the first rush of energy has faded. Highly-spiced foods, coffee, and black tea are some of the things that will leave you feeling energetic, yet often restless and irritable. Most fruits, vegetables and whole grains (unless overeaten) will leave you feeling balanced, calm, clearheaded and relaxed.

If you simply observe how you feel after eating, you will be able to choose your foods accordingly. The signals to look out for are: "fogginess" and difficulty in concentrating after a meal, tiredness, irritability, unexplained emotions and over-reactions. Watch for patterns in these, and try to relate them to your eating. Some such signals may

not appear until the day after you ate whatever caused them. Often, however, the complex combinations of food we eat confuse the issue. We tend to eat lethargy-inducing food along with restless-energy food and often have the illusion of a balanced result. A typical heavy, rich meal followed by coffee, is a good example. In fact, we are simply depleting the body's store of energy, as it struggles to balance these two conflicting inputs. For specific guidance on what foods to avoid combining, see the Food Combination Chart in this section. So, another rule for healthy eating is to keep it simple, especially while you are trying to observe which foods are pleasing and acceptable to your body and which are less so.

This brings us to another difficulty. We tend to eat to please our tongues, rather than to please our whole body-mind. We eat what tempts our palate, in quantities that please our appetite. These preferences, however, are usually stimulated by habit or emotion, rather than by our bodies' true nutritional needs and our digestive and eliminative capacity. These latter messages are more subtle. Yet to eat for health, we need to learn to listen more to the needs of our bodies. Of course, none of us can expect to break these habits overnight. Our awareness and understanding is sure to come faster than our ability or even our desire to change. That's normal. But we can at least begin to balance out our desire and craving-caused choices with consciously-healthful choices. This will be a good start.

FOOD SELECTION GUIDELINES

Foods to Select	Foods to Avoid Whenever Possible
Fresh fruit	Canned or processed foods
Dried fruit	Refined sugar/sugar products
Fresh vegetables	Foods containing preservatives or additives
Sprouted seeds and legumes (alfalfa, lentil, chick pea, sesame, sunflower, peanuts)	Refined flour/flour products
Fruit or vegetable juices	Overcooked foods
Nuts and seeds	Meat, fish and fowl
Milk and dairy products	Animal oils
Beans and legumes	
Whole grains and cereals	*Other non-foods to avoid:*
Whole grain bread	Coffee and teas with caffeine
Honey, molasses, maple syrup	Alcohol
Unprocessed vegetables	Drugs, unless vital
Herbal teas and coffee substitutes	
Tofu and other soy products	
Eggs (in transition diet)	

FASTING

The second stage of purification, as we said earlier, is the elimination of already-existing physical impurities. Vigorous physical exercise has long been recognized as a good way to burn off not only excess calories, but also toxic wastes. Jogging, cycling, regular swimming, racquet sports, yoga and other activities are all excellent ways to exercise the body, and also to rid it of toxic food deposits. Another powerful way to speed up the elimination of toxins is periodic fasting. Fasting is now regaining popular acceptance, after centuries of neglect. In ages past, almost every culture has advocated fasting because of its effectiveness.

"Fasting" can describe many different levels of non-regular eating, not just living on water. It has two major benefits: 1) It gives the digestive system time to rest and repair itself (normally, it works around the clock); and 2) it enables the body to eliminate toxic wastes. Only when the body ceases the digestive process does detoxification occur. Normally, great amounts of body energy (some estimates say up to 65% after a heavy meal) are consumed in digesting our food. A moderately heavy meal requires about 6 hours of work from organs such as the heart, kidneys, and liver; even more from the digestive organs. It takes anywhere from 24-70 hours for one meal to pass right through the body. When we fast, this energy is freed for a thorough housecleaning of the system. The body becomes lighter, more flexible; the mind becomes clearer and more creative. Greater intuitive powers may develop and deep spiritual insights may be experienced after a period of time. A feeling of well-being arises when the energy is freed in this way -- problems suddenly become solutions and ideas flow from nowhere.

The Kripalu Approach advocates a form of fasting adapted from traditional yogic fasting. It involves taking only fruit, fruit juice, or freshly-pressed vegetable juice, for one or more days. We seldom recommend fasting on water alone, as this can cause unpleasant side effects in those not accustomed to fasting. Also, we have found that certain juices, particularly citrus and apple, are very cleansing and yet provide nourishment at the same time. Fresh vegetable juices are even easier for the novice faster; the cleansing is less intense and more nourishment is provided for rebuilding and replacing cells. We generally recommend taking fresh citrus fruit or juice for breakfast, and vegetable juice at lunch and for supper.

Fasting in this way, on a regular basis, definitely leads to greater physical health. One day per week (preferably the same day) is ideal, but if you can't manage that try fasting once every 2, 3, or 4 weeks. From time to time a longer fast is beneficial (3-4 days) particularly at the change of

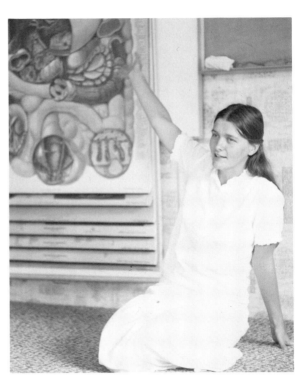

seasons. It will help the body's adaptive processes.

HOW TO DO A SHORT, EASY, ENJOYABLE FAST

PREPARATION

Short fasts are extremely beneficial and not difficult for the person of average health However some factors should be considered such as age, physical condition, weight and the nature of the work which will go on during the fast. An appropriate medical expert should be consulted before young children, underweight people and those with low blood pressure or low blood sugar undertake a fast or purification diet. Also, before attempting a fast of over 5 days, even healthy people should consult a fasting specialist so that they know how to deal with the metabolic changes that may result.

If you are a meat-eater, or if your system is highly toxic, you will find it helpful to prepare for your fast by gradually reducing your intake of meat and substituting a greater variety of wholesome vegetarian foods for a few months. Do this in stages. First, reduce your intake of meat. Then, select one day each week on which you will eat only salad. This will hasten the purification process. Continue with a 1-day salad diet each week for at least eight weeks, and then begin eating fruit one day per week (only one kind of fruit per day). After several weeks of fruit fasting, you will be comfortable graduating to juice.

Eat a light dinner on the evening before a one-day fast. If you plan to fast for more than one day (which is not advised for a first fast) gradually reduce your intake of food over a period of several days before beginning the fast and eat only fruit and salads on the day immediately preceding.

DURING YOUR FAST

Fast on only *one* kind of fruit or fruit juice (rather than combining fruits). Combinations of fruit, such as acid and sweet fruits, do not digest well together and create toxins within the system. Fruits such as apples, grapes and citrus fruits are very cleansing. Bananas are not recommended for fasting, as they are very starchy and not cleansing in nature.

When fasting on juice be sure to drink fresh vegetable juices or pure fruit juices to which no sugar has been added. Fruit juices which are recommended are apple, grape, orange and grapefruit. If the juice is too concentrated for your taste, dilute it with water.

Drink plenty of water throughout the day, as water allows the circulation to flow more freely, thereby accelerating the purification process occurring in the blood and kidneys.

Avoid coffee or caffeine-containing teas. Herbal teas or caffeine-free coffee are fine, but without any sweetener, even honey.

As your body begins to cleanse itself, you may experience some slight discomfort. The pores of your skin will eliminate many toxins, possibly causing body odor. As your lungs eliminate poisons, you may experience bad breath. Your tongue may become coated with a white coating, indicating that cleansing is taking place within your body. (A tongue cleaner is useful at this time. See appendix). In the very early stages of fasting you may experience a slight headache, nausea or cold chills. If these symptoms produce a lot of discomfort, eat a small amount of light food such as a salad, or switch to vegetable juice if you are on fruit juice. Know, however, that these discomforts are a good sign. The more discomfort you feel, the better the fast is working, the more the body is cleansing itself. These symptoms are caused by toxins being poured into your bloodstream, as the result of the increased purification taking place within your body. After some fasting experience, your body will become cleaner and you will be able to fast without any feelings of discomfort or tiredness at all. In fact, as your body purifies, you will gain energy during a fast, particularly after a few days of continuous fasting. You will begin to feel vigorous, energetic, creative, clear, and emotionally balanced.

As a result of fasting, many of the impurities thrown off by the organs are deposited in the intestines. Since your bowel movements will be reduced because you are not taking in any bulk, you need to take special measures to eliminate these impurities. An effective way is to take an enema on the evening of a one-day fast and as needed during longer fasts (see specific instructions later in this chapter). Saunas are also beneficial to facilitate elimination of toxins.

Fast with understanding and awareness of why you are fasting. Keep your mind busy so that it does not dwell on food. If, while fasting, you continually think of foods, you are not fasting but starving, and you will feel deprived and unhappy. Cultivate a positive mental attitude by reading inspiring books and articles about the benefits of fasting (see appendix for suggestions). Direct your awareness to the changes taking place in your body and be happy and proud of what you are doing to purify and rejuvenate your body and to attune more to prana.

EXPERIMENTING WITH A VEGETARIAN DIET

More and more people from all walks of life are discovering the advantages of a vegetarian diet. Many different newspapers and magazines report that athletes say they feel lighter and have more energy on a vegetarian diet, runners claim that they run faster and experience less muscle tension, movie stars find it improves their skin and helps them stay more relaxed, writers and artists say they feel more clear-headed and creative, and many "ordinary" people simply find that they feel better and that it costs less.

Your Ancestors Were Vegetarians

Science is finding increasing evidence that the earliest human beings ate a vegetarian diet, and only turned to meat for survival when their vegetable food sources disappeared. Carnivorous animals have relatively short digestive tracts, and the total time taken for food to move through their entire body is relatively short. Animal flesh putrifies rather rapidly in the warm, moist environment of the body; the rapid digestion and elimination of carnivorous animals prevents this.

Animals which survive on plants have much longer intestinal tracts, to allow for the breakdown of cellulose in the plant matter. Human beings have very long digestive systems -- the intestines alone measure about thirty feet in length! When meat is processed through such a long tract, there is plenty of time for it to putrify and spread toxins throughout the body. Those of us in so-called civilized societies apparently now have such sluggish digestive and eliminative systems that it takes anywhere up to 72 hours for us to process and eliminate our food; in primitive societies the average length of time is 12 to 36 hours, a much healthier time.

Teeth are another indicator of natural diet. Carnivorous animals have sharp, pointed teeth for tearing flesh, whereas vegetarian animals have blunter teeth for grinding. We humans have only two sharp pointed teeth, the "eye teeth". Many scientists feel this is another indication that we began our evolution as vegetarians. Anthropologists examining the teeth of ancient humans by using a recently-discovered and sophisticated method have reported that the pattern of wear on these teeth (as compared to that on animal teeth of the same period) was almost certainly caused by the eating of fruits and vegetables, not meat.

Eating Vegetables is Eating Sunshine

A vegetarian diet is highly suitable for human beings for many other reasons. Vegetables get their energy from the earth, the water and from sunshine. They are high in vitamins and minerals and, as a primary form of food, they can be eaten and digested easily. Meat on the other hand is inefficiently converted from plant life. Its molecules are complex and hard to digest. While meat is high in protein, it is low in many of the vitamins and minerals essential to man.

An increasing number of authorities now believe that many health problems are caused by the toxicity arising from the high uric acid and saturated fat content of meat. Excess uric acid is deposited and accumulated in various organs, causing such diseases as gout and rheumatism. Saturated fats are believed to cause blood pressure problems and hardening of the arteries. Many animals are fed food which has been sprayed with pesticides such as DDT, which are retained in the fatty tissues of the animals and which are then ingested by the people who eat the meat.

Transition Diets

A vegetarian diet is not made up solely of vegetables. It also includes a variety of foods such as fresh fruits, nuts, beans, dairy products and grains. A "pure" vegetarian diet excludes all kinds of meat, fish and poultry, as well as foods containing any form of animal life, even eggs. There are modified vegetarian diets, however, which do include such things as fish and eggs. These are good transition diets for those who have been meat-eaters all of their lives, as it is best not to change to a vegetarian diet suddenly. If you decide you would like to experiment with reducing the meat in your diet, do it gradually, as a sudden change might be a shock to your system.

The most important thing to watch when switching to a vegetarian diet is that you continue to get a balanced diet with ample protein. However recent research is indicating that most Americans do not need nearly as much protein as they are currently getting, or believe they need. Most Americans are eating about 60-70 grams of protein a day, whereas recent studies, supported by historical evidence of other lower protein societies, show that 30-40 is ample.

Vegetarian protein sources are at least the equal of, and some say superior to, animal protein and are easy to include in the average person's diet. Dairy products, whole grains, and seeds and legumes (particularly sprouted ones) are good sources of protein. Soy products are excellent, especially tofu (soy 'cheese', sometimes also called bean curd). There are also some good natural supplements. We particularly recommend brewer's yeast for extra protein and for many of the B-vitamins sometimes lacking in a vegetarian diet, kelp for iodine and trace minerals, and unsulfured blackstrap molasses for iron and minerals.

This is a brief overview of vegetarian eating. Those seriously considering experimenting with a vegetarian diet would do well to read some of the excellent books available on the market (see appendix) and to consult with knowledgeable experts to avoid any stress in transition.

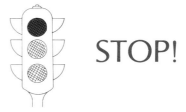

STOP!

STOP! How aware are you of your body's messages *right now*? How are you feeling? Is there tension, stiffness, tiredness in any part of your body? Do you need to get up and stretch? Take some deep breaths? Relax your shoulders? Rest your eyes? Rest your mind? Close your eyes for a minute and take some long, slow deep breaths to enable you to get in touch with your experience. Then respond to what your body is asking you to do.

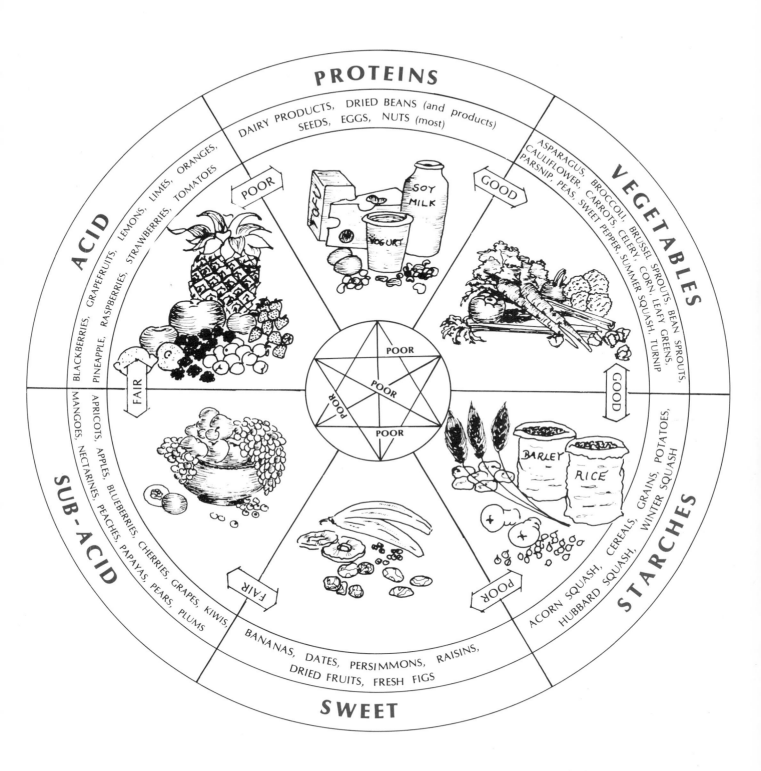

PROTEINS

DAIRY PRODUCTS, DRIED BEANS (and products) SEEDS, EGGS, NUTS (most)

VEGETABLES

ASPARAGUS, BROCCOLI, BRUSSEL SPROUTS, BEAN SPROUTS, CAULIFLOWER, CARROTS, CELERY, CORN, LEAFY GREENS, PARSNIP, PEAS, SWEET PEPPER, SUMMER SQUASH, TURNIP

ACID

BLACKBERRIES, GRAPEFRUITS, LEMONS, LIMES, ORANGES, PINEAPPLE, RASPBERRIES, STRAWBERRIES, TOMATOES

SUB-ACID

APRICOTS, APPLES, BLUEBERRIES, CHERRIES, GRAPES, KIWIS, MANGOES, NECTARINES, PEACHES, PAPAYAS, PEARS, PLUMS

STARCHES

ACORN SQUASH, CEREALS, GRAINS, POTATOES, HUBBARD SQUASH, WINTER SQUASH

SWEET

BANANAS, DATES, PERSIMMONS, RAISINS, DRIED FRUITS, FRESH FIGS

POOR — GOOD — FAIR — GOOD — POOR — FAIR

POOR, POOR, POOR, POOR (center)

SOY MILK — TOFU — YOGURT — BARLEY — RICE

FOOD COMBINING CHART

HOW YOU EAT

Your Habits and Attitudes

Perhaps, like many of us, you know what good, nutritious food is, and yet you still find yourself sometimes eating "junk foods", overeating, eating too fast, eating wrong combinations and getting indigestion...and you wonder "Why? Why, when I know better, do I still have these poor eating habits?" The following article by Yogi Amrit Desai will give you a part of the answer. The rest of the answer is unique to you and will have to come from your own self-analysis and observation.

EATING CONSCIOUSLY

by Yogi Amrit Desai

How Relaxation Affects Appetite

A major cause of inappropriate eating is hidden tension. Whenever you experience unpleasant emotions or feel tense, you are losing prana, or energy. Then you unconsciously feel the need to replace this lost energy by eating.

Unfortunately, when you don't eat wisely, you lose more energy processing the food than you gain from the food, and so a low-energy cycle is created. This cycle can be broken at several places. First, if you learn to be more relaxed you will need less food, because there is less lost energy to be replenished. When you are very tense, you may eat 3 or 4 large meals a day and still feel hungry. Yet, if you are relaxed, one or two light meals may be sufficient. Second, you can improve your eating patterns, so that digestion does not drain the energy you gained from the food. And third, you can understand and change the tension-related attitudes that affect your eating habits.

When we are tense, we tend to seek relaxation and fulfillment through gratifying our senses. Food is our fastest and easiest way to do this. Actually, our search for pleasure and enjoyment through food, entertainment, fun and sexual relationships, is often hiding an inner emptiness that comes from spiritual starvation -- from not feeling fulfilled on all levels of our being. But we usually recognize only the physical lack of fulfillment. Western society is very food-oriented, with associated problems of overeating, poor digestion, etc. Television advertising reflects this very accurately. Commercials for delicious-looking foods are almost immediately followed by commercials for antacids and digestive aids, or for the latest fad in reducing diets!

Rediscovering Natural Hunger

Because of this excessive food orientation, and the constant seeking of taste-sensations to satisfy ourselves superficially and dull our inner yearnings, we have overstimulated our appetites to the point where we can no longer hear the real inner physical needs of our bodies or prana. Instead, the appetite we hear and respond to is the one produced by our minds and our desires for taste sensations. These desires are simply repetitions of previous experiences; habits based on memories of previously pleasurable tastes. And so we have developed eating habits which detract from, rather than contribute to, our health and well-being.

Quite often, we eat when we are not even really hungry, in the sense of having a naturally-stimulated physical hunger. You know from experience that when you have been physically very active and out in the fresh air, you have such a healthy appetite that even the simplest foods taste wonderfully satisfying. But when you have been sitting at a desk all day in a busy office, even the most delicious meal may not fully satisfy you. When we cannot experience the complete satisfaction that comes from eating with natural hunger, we often seek artificial ways to gain that satisfaction. We eat foods which are elaborately prepared, exotic and rich, with unusual tastes, exciting colors and textures. We try to stimulate hunger, artificially, with little "appetizers" and a variety of alcoholic "aperitifs" (the word actually means appetite-stimulant). Of course, neither the additives that are needed to create these foods nor the alcohol contribute to health. Satisfaction comes from how much genuine hunger we experience, not from the elaborate taste or texture of what we consume. This loss of natural hunger is the cause of most overeating too. When we are tense, we are not able to enjoy our lives fully, and so we seek pleasure from eating. But because of our unhealthy, physically-inactive lifestyle, we cannot derive full satisfaction from the food we eat, and so we seek that satisfaction by eating more and more, creating another endless unhealthy cycle.

Eat To Live -- Or Live To Eat?

At the root of the problem lies the fact that many people have forgotten the true role of eating in life. Eating is first of all to provide nourishment and sustain our life processes so that we can explore and develop our higher potentials. Instead, we have distorted the basic function of food and made it primarily a means to satisfy our senses of taste and smell. If we forget this primary purpose of eating, if we consume food that is basically healthy, we will still be likely to damage our health by overeating or combining our foods unwisely. What is available in health food stores today is ready proof of this. These stores are full of a broad selection of "natural", "healthy", "organic" delicacies and treats, all packaged to tempt the palate! So you still run the danger of over-indulging, overeating or eating poorly, even with health foods, unless you remain conscious of your true purpose in eating. You must eat to nourish your body, because it is, as many sages have said, the "temple of the soul".

Remember that "natural" does not necessarily mean "best". Even natural foods need to be eaten with discrimination. Base your diet in accordance with what you know from experience is best for your own health. Eat in accordance with your prana. Most of all, become conscious of your motivations for eating. As you cultivate attitudes toward eating which are more supportive of your health, they will yield immediate benefits; you will both enjoy your food more, and gain a richer experience of health and well-being in your life.

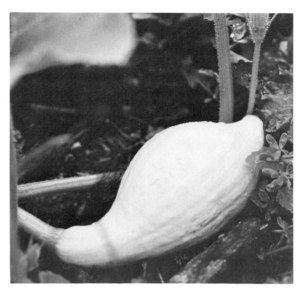

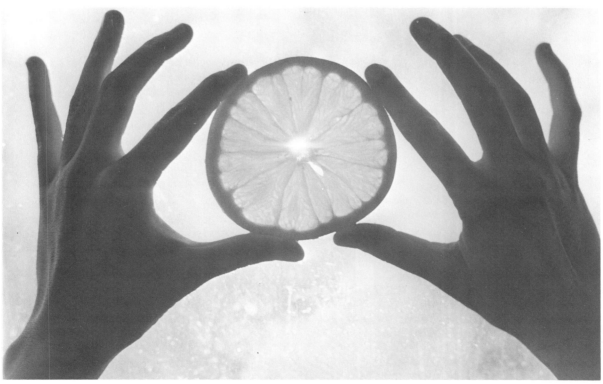

HOW TO CULTIVATE THE ART OF CONSCIOUS EATING

What does conscious eating mean? It means eating with full awareness of where, how and why, as well as what, you are eating. It means slowing down and paying attention -- really being there. It means devoting your full attention, during a meal, to the actual eating process, so as to obtain both maximum health benefits *and* maximum enjoyment. Here's how to cultivate this art:

1. Eat only when you are hungry. Even if you eat more than someone else, it will benefit you as long as you are hungry. If you do not get much joy out of eating, if you are dissatisfied with the variety of food available, you are either not really hungry or you are eating more than your natural appetite requires. When you are hungry, the simplest food tastes the most delicious. After eating, you should feel relaxed and alert. If you feel tired or sluggish, you will know that you have eaten too much. When you eat less, you may experience hunger at first. This is because any change from habit will give rise to an initial protest from the body, but this protest comes from the previous times that you have overeaten or eaten improperly, not from having missed a meal or two. The initial discomfort which comes from getting to know true hunger is caused by the body beginning to purify. This purification is a positive, healthy process.

Hunger is a gift of nature. It is an expression of prana, our inner physician. When you allow yourself to become truly hungry, then eating is an exquisite pleasure, a natural fulfillment of a real bodily need. Let your prana tell you when to eat, what to eat, and how much to eat. Because each person is different, no one can prescribe what is best for someone else. Each person has his or her own natural needs. Discovering these needs will bring a new health and vitality to your life. Only when you allow yourself to experience real hunger and discover the natural rhythm of your own bodily needs will you experience the real joy of eating.

2. Eat regularly at specific times. Plan each meal and eat a quantity such that you will again be hungry by the time of your next meal. In this way, you will eat only when you are hungry and you will eat regularly as well.

3. Focus all your attention on what is happening in your mouth as you chew. This has two benefits. First, you will chew thoroughly. This is important because a significant portion of the digestive process is accomplished by enzymes secreted in the mouth. If you do not chew properly, you are bypassing this important stage of digestion and forcing your stomach to compensate by working

harder than nature intended. Chronic indigestion, gas and constipation will result. Second, if you really pay attention to your chewing, you will gain such taste satisfaction from your food that you will not need to overeat.

4. Select the proper amount and type of food for your individual system. This will vary according to your age, weight, sex and the type of work you do. Strenuous physical work requires a heavier diet; sedentary work is done more efficiently when eating lightly.

5. Avoid eating when you are angry, excited, tense, depressed, sick, hurried, or tired. Wait until your mind becomes calm and your natural hunger returns. The hunger you experience when tense is not true hunger. It is mentally-induced hunger, designed to provide a nervous outlet for your anxieties. True hunger arises only when you are relaxed.

6. Always eat in a pleasant atmosphere. Make your meals attractive and your place of eating pleasant and soothing. Begin your meal with a simple prayer or by observing a moment of silence to reflect with gratitude upon the gift of life which comes to you through food. A prayerful attitude relaxes you, prepares your digestive system to more fully assimilate the food you eat, and enables you to draw more prana from your food.

7. When you are eating - EAT! Try not to talk, read, listen to the radio, watch TV, etc. Silence is important because it prevents the mental disturbances which can easily arise in the course of conversation. Conversation and other activities distract you from the awareness that it is necessary to chew food properly and taste it fully. When you talk, read, etc., your body must work harder to derive maximum benefit from the food. When you do need to talk, make sure your conversation is gentle, pleasant and loving.

8. Make eating an act of meditation, an act of reverence for your body and your inner self. Be fully aware of what is occurring within your body. Visualize your digestive process and feel that the food is being converted into pranic energy for the sustenance of your body, mind and spirit.

9. If you overeat, accept yourself! You probably will overeat at times and that's natural. Learning to eat consciously happens gradually, so that there will be occasions when you forget or choose not to pay attention to your body's needs and, instead, listen to the mind's artificial demands. The most important thing at such times is to accept yourself and not create emotional tension and guilt about having eaten too much. Emotional reactions to eating will do more harm than the overeating itself. What's more, they will probably lead to more overeating, because they create tension in you. So if you overeat, don't worry about it. Learn from your experience; try to examine what led to your overeating and correct the conditions for the next time.

In summary, for better overall health of body, mind, emotions and spirit, eat consciously. Start by simplifying your diet, learn to become aware of how different foods affect your energy and consciousness, and begin to purify your system through more exercise and moderate fasting (one day a week is very helpful, but even once a month will be good). And always remember: balance and patience are the keys. Recognize and accept that it may take time to change ingrained habits and remember that diet and nutrition are only one of the 8 ways to health.

So, take it easy and love yourself!

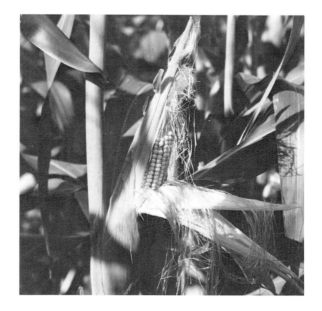

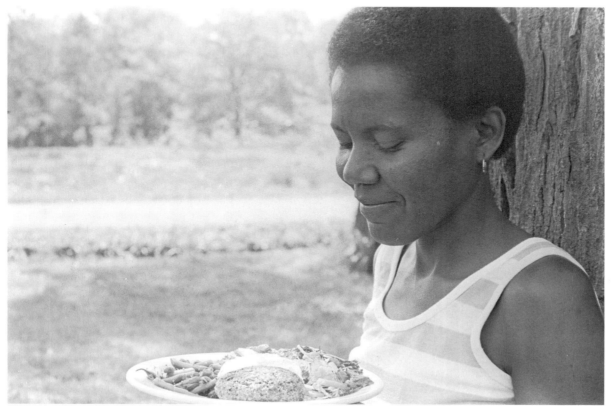

OTHER HEALTH TOOLS TO TRY

Colon Cleansing Through Enemas and Colonics

The Kripalu Center for Holistic Health offers both colonic irrigation therapy and instruction in self-administered enemas, as a part of the overall cleansing and purification of the body required for Holistic Health.

The History

Colonic cleansing, in one form or another, has a venerable history. Over 6,000 years ago, the earliest yogis experienced an automatic process called "basti" occurring as their bodies were spontaneously purified by their practices.

When their bodies were immersed in water, spontaneous muscular contractions occurred, drawing water into the colon to cleanse it. This became one of the formalized cleansing techniques of yoga known as kriyas. People of many other lands have developed methods of cleaning out the intestines through more mechanical means.

The Benefits

Many years of observing the experiences of hundreds of residents and visitors have led us to believe that some form of colonic cleansing is highly desirable at different stages on the path to greater health. There is a factor in disease that yogis and ancient healers have known experientially for thousands of years. This is that much illness and disease, particularly chronic, is a result of general toxemia (toxic blood), which begins in the colon where uneliminated food wastes remain trapped and become bonded with mucus, forming an encrustation. Beneficial bacteria are destroyed as their environment is polluted, and as putrefaction sets in toxic bacteria are released. These are absorbed through the intestinal walls into the bloodstream, are circulated in the body, and begin to cause disease and degeneration of healthy body tissues. The colon, encrusted as it is, loses its elasticity and ability to undergo peristalsis, thereby further slowing down the elimination of wastes. The longer waste products remain in the body, the more putrefaction and resulting toxic products are created. This causes further degeneration of muscle tone in the colon, and so a vicious cycle is set up.

What is the original cause of colon problems? There are many. Most experts believe that our present day diet of over-refined, chemical-laden food and our habit of taking laxatives are major causative factors, along with the extreme tensions experienced in our present day, fast-moving society. Whatever the cause, the results are tangible and experiential. Many Americans suffer from some form of eliminative disorders, usually chronic constipation. The healthy body should, ideally, have a bowel movement after each meal, and food should pass through the body within about 24 hours. Most people experience fewer bowel movements than that, and it may take anywhere up to 72 hours for the complete ingestion-elimination process.

Even if we are not suffering from any apparent digestive problems, it is estimated that most Americans carry up to 5-10 pounds of encrusted, hardened feces lining their colons, inhibiting the body's ability to fully absorb the nutrients in food. Enemas and colonics help with removal of this. The usual experience is one of an instant sense of well-being and greater vitality, and health, even among those who are not actually sick.

THE METHOD

[1] Colonics

Colonic irrigation therapy, if performed by a skilled technician, is the best method for cleaning the colon because it can send the liquid high up into the intestines where an enema cannot reach. Colonic lavage consists of having the colon filled with and washed by a constant stream of water fed by a carefully controlled machine. A recent innovation is the use of highly oxygenated water (this is the type of treatment provided by the Kripalu Center for Holistic Health). This is the optimum method, for the added oxygen not only facilitates the cleansing but also acts as a healing agent and stimulates rapid replacement of the beneficial bacteria necessary for efficient digestion and elimination.

Gradually, over a series of colonic treatments, the old, encrusted and putrifying feces are dislodged from the intestinal walls and washed out, and the colon is freed and stimulated to perform more efficiently. The source of blood toxicity is thus removed, and better health results, often rapidly and seemingly miraculously.

Until recently, there has been no professional training or certification for colonic administrators, and not all those who offer the service are adequately skilled or even informed. Shop carefully!

[2] Enemas

An enema is a self-administered, simpler form of "colonic irrigation" (colon washing). Usually, it consists of suspending a special, flexible bag of water (or other liquid) 2 or 3 feet above the buttocks and allowing it to gently flow into the body, in slow stages. Even a "high enema" cannot reach as high as a mechanic "colonic" nor, of course, can oxygenated water be administered.

Nevertheless, experience shows that simple enemas, if taken with skilled guidance, greatly reduce toxicity and facilitate elimination, reducing constipation. Enemas are particularly helpful at the onset of colds, flu, etc. and can sometimes even eliminate the toxicity which made one susceptible to the attack from germs or viruses. They are also excellent while fasting (we would even say indispensable on longer fasts).

HOW TO TAKE AN ENEMA

1. Obtain an enema bag (most drug stores carry them, and the cost is minimal) and an 18-inch catheter tube.

2. Find a suitable, quiet bathroom and toilet where you can remain undisturbed for 30-45 minutes and where you can lie down comfortably.

3. Fill the enema bag with 1-2 quarts of warm-tepid water (body temperature) or other liquid (see below), and suspend it 2-3 feet above the ground. Allow the liquid to flow out from the bag for 2-3 seconds to remove any air bubbles.

4. Lubricate the nozzle and your anus with a little vegetable oil and assume a comfortable position. Various positions are possible, and the ultimate choice is personal. We recommend either:

a) lying on your side, with your knees slightly bent: first lying on the left side, then the back, then the right. Draw your right knee up to your chest, while retaining the water.
b) kneeling on all fours.
c) lying on the back with hips raised by a small pillow, some towels, etc.

You may assume whichever position feels most comfortable to you and allows the best flow. You will probably want to vary it.

5. Now insert the nozzle.

6. Gently controlling the flow with the clip, slowly allow it to trickle into your colon. You will experience the **desire to** evacuate from time to time, but unless there is real pain or cramping, resist the urge as long as you can. Stopping the flow and massaging the colon will help eliminate the air pockets that can cause discomfort.

7. Ideally, work towards holding the liquid for a period of 10 to 20 minutes (more or less, depending on the liquid). At first you will be able to hold only very little water, for a very short period of time. With practice, you will be able to hold more and longer.

After you hold and expel several small quantities, you may refill the bag. You will be able to hold more as you evacuate more waste. It is important to be gentle, yet firm with your body. Try not to evacuate as soon as you feel the urge, but avoid forcing or straining your body.

WHAT LIQUID SHOULD I USE?

1. Water (warm, not hot.)

2. Lemon water (just a small quantity of freshly strained lemon juice added; 3-4 tsp. per 2 quarts).

3. Weak camomile tea or comfrey tea (helps eliminate mucus).

There are many other more or less exotic mixtures that can be used for specific purposes, but these should be advised and supervised by a Holistic Health specialist.

CAUTION

Those with any kind of colon disease should first consult a specialist with a background in enemas and colonics, before attempting an enema or colonic irrigation.

Also, it is quite easy to become "addicted" to enemas as either a substitute for laxatives or for proper eating. Enemas are for occasional purification or crisis intervention and should not become habitual, as they may destroy muscle tone in the intestines or create other complications.

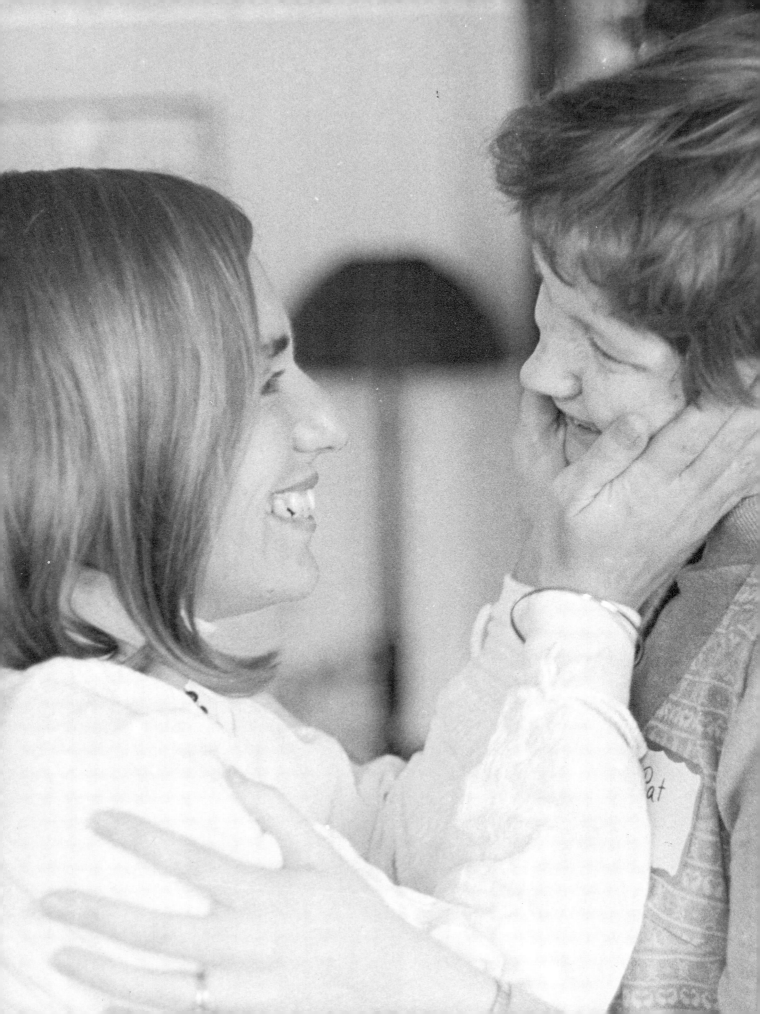

WAY SIX
communication and self-expression

THE IMPORTANCE OF COMMUNICATION

How many people do you communicate with in an average day? Probably dozens; hundreds in a week, thousands in a year, and who knows how many in a lifetime. From the most casual and superficial transaction to the most intimate human relationship, our moments are filled with communications. They are the very lifeblood of our existence as social beings. Our methods of communicating have evolved tremendously over the centuries since the first ape man grunted to his neighbor. Language slowly evolved, then languages, then written forms, from primitive picture-alphabets through cuneiform script to the present day simplified letter alphabets of the West. The history of communication is the history of civilization.

The invention of printing was the beginning trickle of non-interpersonal communications, which has grown to a flood in our century. The potential for one person's ideas to influence many was opened up and mankind entered a new phase of communications. The twentieth century has seen an explosion of communications systems, from typewriter to tape recorder, from wireless to video, from advertising to xerox machines. We are awash, it seems, in a sea of machines. Our eyes and ears are bombarded day long, and often night long, with messages. Where once communication was a simple phenomenon of one person

talking or signaling to another, now we are all intercepting (willingly or otherwise) millions of messages to and from everyone in society. Our communication-bearing techniques and technologies have become increasingly sophisticated. More messages can be carried farther and faster to more people and more far-flung locations than ever before in history.

More Is Not Better

The question is, has the *quality* of our communication improved along with the *quantity*? Do we communicate, on the person-to-person level, better, or only more and faster? Has the communications explosion helped us to understand each other better, as human beings, or are we drowning in a self-inflicted flood of messages? Is the noise of our words deafening us? How has the growth of communication affected our present-day consciousness? Have we become so skilled at exchanging messages (facts, opinions, theories) that we have overlooked the exchange of real feelings? Can we really express ourselves? Do we know how to listen?

The efficiency of message delivery systems (books, film, television, advertising etc.) is at an all time high. There is a "communications industry", with "professional communicators" and "communications experts." There are degrees offered in communications. Yet still we find that true understanding between one individual and

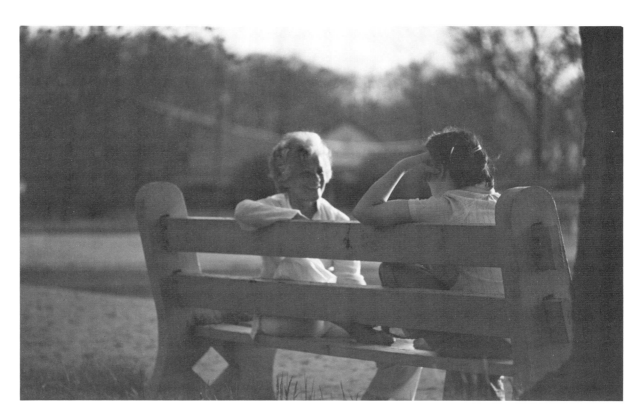

another is blocked by "communication problems." Marriages flounder and nations go to war because of communication breakdowns.

In our daily lives, every little interaction we have with another human being is a communication. As such, it has the potential to draw us closer in love and understanding (and thus to take a small step in drawing all the people of the world closer) or to increase the gulf between us. Even a simple transaction with a clerk in a store can make or mar both our day and theirs, and interactions with our loved ones and co-workers are, of course, much more intensely potent. We have experienced that few things feel better than being understood by (or truly understanding) another human being. Yet still we encounter difficulties.

What is it that blocks true communication between people? How can we learn to overcome these blocks? How can we improve our communication skills? What is the secret of good communication?

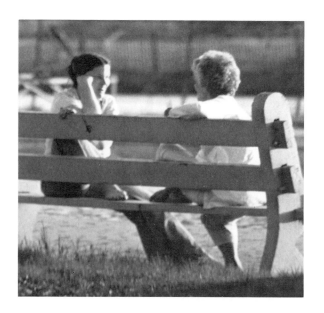

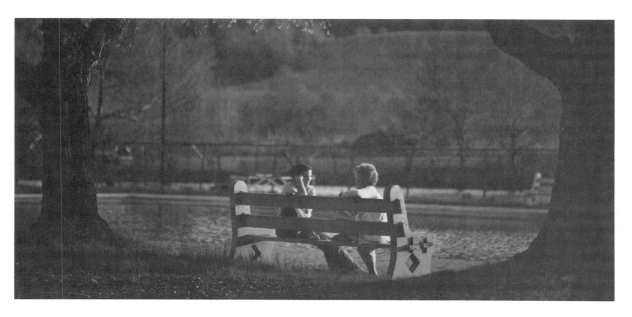

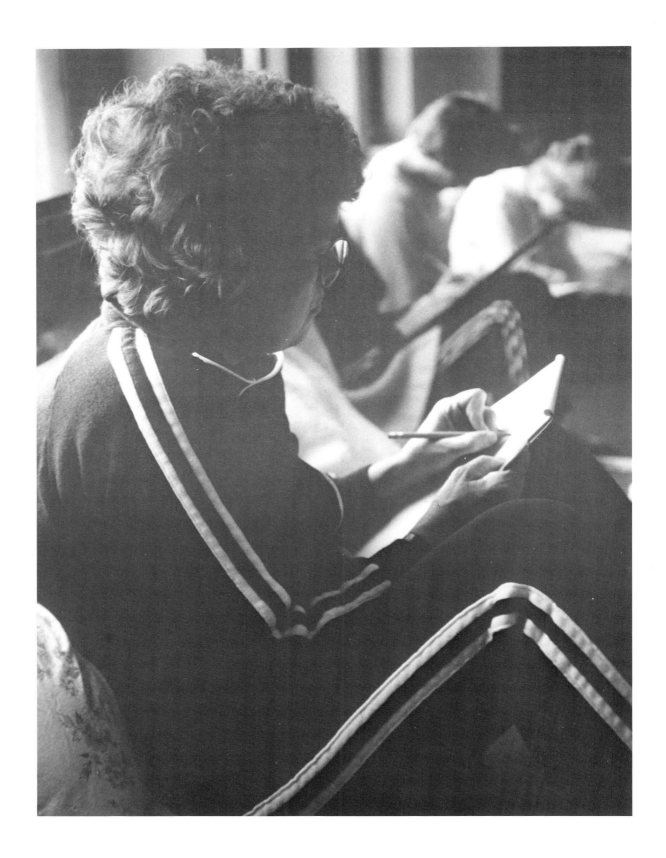

Self-Discovery Experience 13

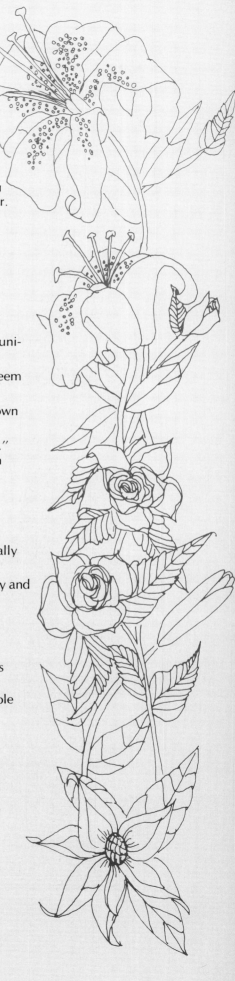

How Well Do You Communicate?

Before reading further, complete this Self-Discovery Experience to see where you stand and to gain an experiential basis for understanding the material in this chapter.

Note: Some questions are worded in a very similar way, yet are quite different in meaning. Be sure to answer exactly what is asked.

Before writing your answer to each question, close your eyes, relax, and allow the answers to filter up to you from your unconscious, without mentally censoring the feelings and intuitions that emerge.

Awareness

1. Write down some brief sentences using the words "communication" and "communicate" in as many different ways as you can, to illustrate their range of meanings.

2. Look over what you have written, and summarize briefly what these two words seem to mean for you.

3. See if you can think of any other meanings you may have missed and jot them down too.

4. Reflect for a moment on how you *feel* when you hear the word "communication." What associations does it bring up for you? What images? What emotions? Jot them down.

5. Now complete the following sentences:

(a) My communications with other people are usually…

(b) I feel my ability to communicate with other people is…

(c) When I have had a good clear communication with someone, I feel (emotionally and physically)…

(d) When I am involved in a mis-communication of some kind, I feel (emotionally and physically)…

(e) When I am involved in a mis-communication with someone else, it is usually because…

(f) I think that most misunderstandings between people are caused by…

(g) When I do have a clear, harmonious communication with another person, it is because…

(h) I think that I personally would be able to communicate better with other people if…

(i) What I would most like to learn about communication is…

Acceptance and Adjustment: First read the material which follows.

COMMUNICATIONS AND YOUR HEALTH

Have you ever stopped to consider the hidden messages behind some of our more common idiomatic expressions? Reflect for a moment on what these familiar phrases are saying: "He's a real pain in the neck!" "I had to eat my words!" "I had to bite back what I was going to say." "I really cannot stomach that woman!" "I'll just have to shoulder the responsibility." "He is positively guilt-ridden." "I swallowed my humiliation." "He has a stiff upper lip approach to life."

There are many such others. What they indicate is a close link between how we express ourselves and how we feel physically. They also demonstrate very clearly that when we are not able to express what we are feeling, or to interact harmoniously with others on the spoken level, there is a blockage in our flow of energy, a holding down or in of our prana. Communication is the external expression of our energy, of who we are. How we express ourselves, how this expression is received by others, and how we feel about our ability to communicate are key factors in our experience of health. Communication is particularly important in the holistic interpretation of health, because it looks at the well-being of the whole person, not just the physical body.

What do we mean when we use the words "communication" and "communicate?" Probably your definition included some of the following: to tell, to explain, to express an opinion, to convey facts, to make someone understand something, or simply to talk. All these meanings are correct, but they are incomplete if they make the assumption that all communication requires two people. A basic dictionary definition "to communicate" is "to impart or exchange knowledge," yet it also includes the definition "to make known", and this making known can happen within the individual. We need to make our feelings known to ourselves on an inner level as well as to communicate them to others. There is a second possible mis-apprehension about communication that needs to be clarified before we go further. This is that "to communicate", in a two-person exchange, means to be the speaker -- I communicate something to you and then you communicate something back to me. This assumes that speaking is an active process which requires energy, and listening is a passive process, which doesn't.

First, Learn to Communicate with Yourself

In this chapter, we will begin by looking at the idea that communication is an internal, as well as, and even before, it is an external process. Yogi Desai says: "Until you *first* learn to communicae with yourself, you cannot hope to communicate effectively with others." We have all had experiences which backed up this statement, if we reflect for a moment. Remember those times

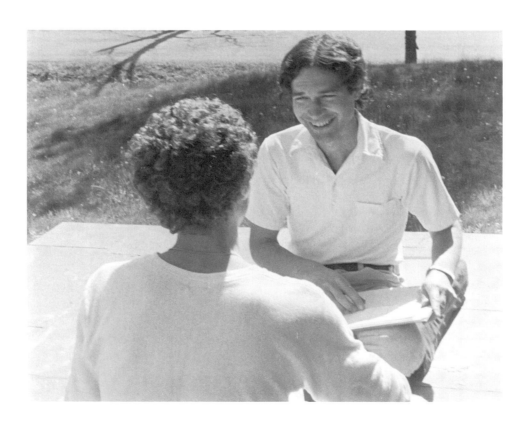

when you had to give up explaining something in frustration because you realized that you weren't sure of what it was that you *really* wanted to say.

This chapter is divided into two sections. In the first we will look at communicating with yourself as a first step to better communications with others. In the second section we will look at a concept called "Active Listening," a type of listening which requires as much energy and attention as speaking, if not more. Until each one of the many voices inside us is heard and understood by others, we cannot hope to communicate effectively. Until we can put as much energy and love into listening to others as we do into expressing our own points of view and feelings, we will not make others feel really heard either, and true communication will not happen.

COMMUNICATION SKILLS I: SELF—EXPRESSION

You Don't Understand Me Because I'm Afraid To Tell You Who I Am

Communication is a process that happens on two levels: the level of experience and the level of expression. The first level concerns our communication with ourselves; the second, our communication with others. Both are equally important. Our feelings are at the core of our experience of life; our communication with others is essential for our survival in the world and for our sense of connection with our fellow human beings.

Miscommunication or poor communication with others is a common experience. It is at the heart of most of our difficulties with other people. Miscommunication with ourselves (our lack of ability to understand what is really going on inside of us) often is at the root of any tension or discomfort we may feel. Even if we feel that we already communicate well with those around us, a deeper understanding of our inner communications system will yield great benefits in the form of a more harmonious, flowing and loving life.

The Missing Link

How do these internal and external communications problems arise? There is a missing link in our personal communications "network" -- something that we frequently overlook, and yet which is responsible for most of our communication problems. This missing link is what happens to our feelings in the time *between* their organization and their expression. Most of us have difficulty expressing our feelings at one time or another, yet we are often not aware of the true reason for this. When we prepare to express ourselves, a complex chain of events happens inside of us. It occurs so fast that we are usually not

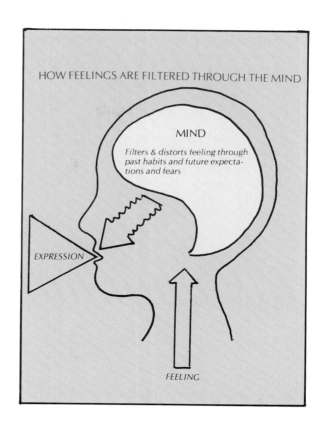

HOW FEELINGS ARE FILTERED THROUGH THE MIND

MIND

Filters & distorts feeling through past habits and future expectations and fears

EXPRESSION

FEELING

conscious of its existence. This chain of inner events (which will be discussed) results in a distortion of our original feeling, our authentic experience.

It is difficult to express feelings, which are non-verbal, non-conceptual, in the form of language, which must necessarily work through words and concepts. To this difficulty we then add that of trying to express something which we ourselves do not really understand, because we have lost touch with the original basic feelings which motivated us to speak.

What we are conscious of wanting to express is often quite different from what we originally felt. Feelings occur first in the body, and our body then manifests the effects of those feelings. When what we eventually try to express is something different, a split occurs between body and mind, feeling and expression. This split results in physical tension and emotional frustration at our inability to express what we are experiencing, and feelings of lack of love because the other person does not understand what we are trying to say. Really it is we, ourselves, who do not know what we are trying to say, because we no longer know what it is we were feeling. Yet we are not aware that we do not know. We believe we are simply unable to express what we feel.

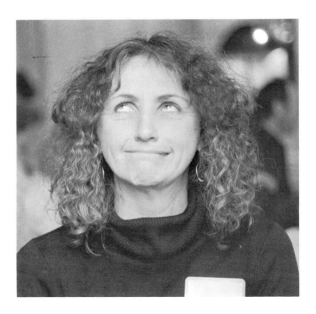

Bridging the Gap Between Feeling and Expression

In order to remedy the situation, we need to be able to bridge that gap between feeling and expression. To do this we must understand the unconscious internal process that distorts our feelings even before we recognize them consciously and try to express them.

This distortion is caused by a negative intervention of the mind. It is, of course, necessary for us to use our minds to integrate our feelings and our experiences into our lives. The proper role of the mind is to note, consciously and objectively, what we are feeling and experiencing in our bodies, interpret what this means in positive terms of our needs to interact with the outside world, and then provide us with the words we need to carry out that interaction.

The Mind as Distorting Filter

Unfortunately, this mental process has become distorted. The original cause of this distortion is fear, but we do not recognize it as such because it has grown habitual over the years. Our minds are no longer able to perceive our feelings objectively and focus them clearly. The mind has acquired the qualities of a filter over the years, transmitting only a part of the light of our feelings. Or we could compare the mind to a distorting lens, which bends the rays of light of our feelings as they pass through, and makes them unrecognizable. This distorting lens or mental filter is composed of two major elements: our habit patterns and our desires and expectations for the future. We want to control the present and the future, so that they

turn out differently than our memories of unsuccessful past experiences. We are constantly, yet unconsciously, using the present to right the unremembered wrongs of the past. Our past is an unfinished Gestalt, an incomplete circle we are trying to complete. So each attempt at communication in the present is an unconscious attempt to achieve a communication we didn't achieve in the past (or that we believe, subconsciously, that we didn't achieve). This has come about in the following way. As small children, we naturally and spontaneously expressed our feelings as they arose. We had no verbal ability, and so we did not try to translate them into words. If you watch small children, you will see this. Joy, anger, pain, hunger, all are expressed spontaneously through the body (laughter, shouts, tears) and all pass quickly and are forgotten. There is no inhibition, no holding back. As we grew older we began to find, to our shocked surprise, that some of these spontaneous expressions of feeling were no longer acceptable; they were considered childish, negative or inappropriate to mature, civilized human beings. We learned it was "bad" to express anger by striking or shouting. We were told not to cry, because only babies (or girls) cry. We were made to control our hunger until it was time to eat or to ask for food rather than cry for it. Because of our need for approval, one of the deepest of human needs, we learned to fear the expression of our feelings, to inhibit and mask them, even to feel guilty about having them at all.

From Mask to Mask

As we learned to express ourselves through language, we struggled to find words which would express our feelings in a way that was acceptable to the powerful adults in our lives: our parents, our teachers. We began to wear masks, to disguise our true feelings from others and to protect ourselves from criticism and disapproval. Gradually, over time, we forgot that we were wearing a mask. As the song says: "When I fool the people I fear, I fool myself as well." The internal process of fear and denial of our true feelings happened so fast that we quickly became unaware of it. It passed into our personality as a mechanical, habitual inner process. And so we became distant from ourselves -- living once-removed from our real experience. But one denial and removal gradually necessitated another, and then another. It is like lying; one lie requires another to cover it up, and another to cover up the second one, and so on. We were constantly putting on a new mask to cover up the old one, when we feared that it had become unacceptable.

Believing In Our Own Pretense

In order to become acceptable to others, and to gain their approval, we pretended to be different than we were. We ended up believing in our own pretense, in order to make sense of our inner universe. This is illustrated by a psychological theory called "cognitive dissonance." This states that when we hold two contradictory cognitions, or perceptions, about our environment, our subconscious mind distorts one of these perceptions in order to eliminate the mental dissonance (the disharmony) which results. Such is our unconscious drive for inner consistency. The mind will spontaneously and unconsciously lie to itself in order to produce agreement between two discordant elements. This is what happens in our communication system. "If I want to be accepted, I must be a good person. A good person is not supposed to feel angry. So, I am not angry." is the syllogism that develops. The intermediate step of "I will not *show* anger" is often unconsciously omitted.

Ironically enough, we begin our self-deception out of a fear of being rejected, and we end up experiencing rejection anyway, not because we are angry but because we are not expressing our real feelings. We are not "being real". Other people are subtly able to feel that we are not being real with them, even if they don't interpret that feeling consciously.

So we go around wearing masks -- rejecting ourselves, and rejecting each other -- all because we have allowed our fear of rejection, which may have been an illusion at the beginning, to habitually distort who we are and who we say we are. We are, once again , trapped in a vicious cycle.

The results of this vicious cycle are profound. Not only are we unable to communicate clearly with others, but we have lost the ability to communicate clearly with ourselves. We no longer know what it is we are really feeling. We no longer know who we really are. The gap between our feeling, our thinking and our action is so wide, that we are like different people trapped in the same body.

Accepting Our Feelings As They Are

How do we solve this problem? First, by beginning to observe ourselves closely in order to see where it is that we deny our original feeling out of fear, how we distort it, and what is the result. We must bring the whole unconscious, mechanical process under the spotlight of our consciousness. Then, in order to be able to view our feelings objectively, with clarity, we must be willing to let go both of the fear of others' rejection anc of our own self-rejection. We must accept our feelings as they *are*. This does not necessarily mean that we have to express them -- that is a different matter. But we do need to recognize, without guilt, that this is a perfectly natural, human response. Only then, when we have become clear about what we are really feeling and have accepted it, can we communicate clearly with other people.

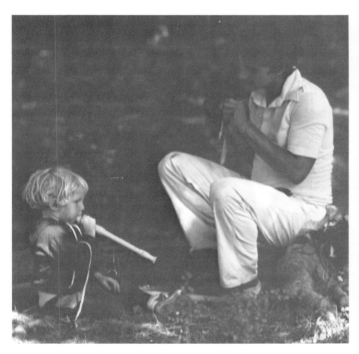
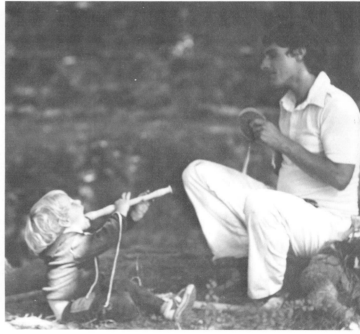

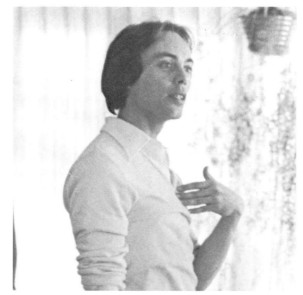

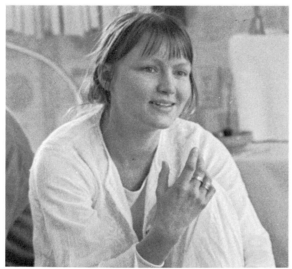

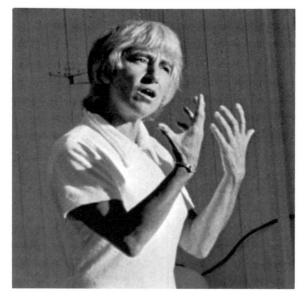

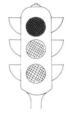

STOP!

STOP! How aware are you of your body's messages *right now*? How are you feeling? Is there tension, stiffness, tiredness in any part of your body? Do you need to get up and stretch? Take some deep breaths? Relax your shoulders? Rest your eyes? Rest your mind? Close your eyes for a minute and take some long, slow deep breaths to enable you to get in touch with your experience. Then respond to what your body is asking you to do.

Self-Discovery Experience

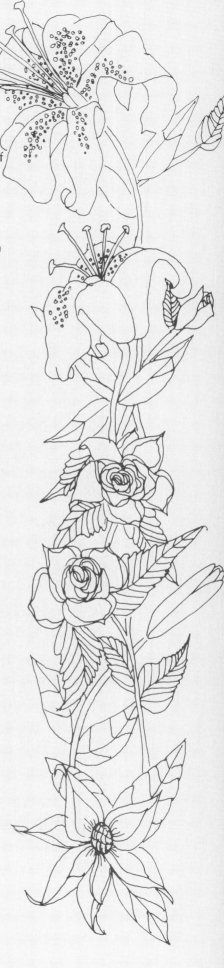

Acceptance

Review the answers to the questions in the Awareness section (p. 143). Read them as if they were written by someone else, and you were being asked to evaluate them. As a detached observer, look for and write down:

1. Patterns that you see you have in communications problems.

2. Your strengths in communicating with others.

3. Your greatest areas of weakness. For example: Do you feel easily frustrated when you are not understood? Do you feel inadequate and unable to express yourself in certain situations? Are you at ease in communicating facts, figures and opinions, but insecure in talking about your own emotions and feelings?

4. Your "blind spots" in communications. Do you tend to blame others for communications difficulties, or to retreat into "shyness" to avoid situations?

5. Any other observations that occur to you that may be helpful.

Remember to maintain an objectivity about your observations, without feeling any sense of inadequacy. Accept that everyone has some difficulty and you are no different. Language is, at best, an approximation of what is going on inside us.

Adjustment

1. Write down some specific areas that you would like to work on in improving your communication skills.

2. As you go through the rest of this chapter, make notes as you encounter further areas on which you want to work.

Having understood and accepted that the first step in good external communications is to have good internal communications, the question becomes: "How can I learn to understand my inner communication problems more clearly?" Here are two techniques to meet that need. The first is a form of introspection which follows the 3A's format. It outlines the questions you need to ask yourself in order to become clear about your own part in a specific situation of miscommunication or conflict. Very often, if you are able to formulate the right questions to ask yourself, you will find the seeds of the answers in the questions themselves.

The second technique is one you can use ongoingly to help yourself clarify the feelings, awarenesses and observations that come up on a daily basis. It takes the form of a written communications journal -- one with a special format to help you gain insights and see patterns in what you record.

HOW TO IMPROVE YOUR INTERNAL COMMUNICATIONS THROUGH INTROSPECTION

Whenever you have a conflict with someone else, carefully examine the situation in an honest and open way, when you are no longer feeling any of the strong emotions that were present in the situation itself. The following exercise has helped many people to resolve conflicts with others and within themselves. Using this method will help to increase your understanding, enhance your inner harmony, and make your communication with those around you more effective.

- Begin by relaxing your body and mind as you close your eyes and take a few long deep breaths.

- Choose a situation of conflict you would like to understand more clearly and use for your growth. Resolve to seek the lesson for you in that situation in an honest and open manner.

- Write down your answers to the following questions and statements as clearly and objectively as you can:

1) Describe what happened.
2) Ask "What did I..
   ...think?
   ...feel?
   ...do?
   ...say?
3) Now as honestly and completely as you can, put yourself in the other person's place. Ask: "What did he/she
   ...think?
   ...feel?
   ...do?
   ...say?

4) What did I want from the situation? What did he/she want?

5) In every situation of conflict, there is some underlying fear on both sides. Ask yourself "What were the fears in this situation? What was I afraid of deep down? What was I afraid would or would not happen?"

6) Now, taking all the above into consideration, what was the effect of my action(s) on
   ...the other person?
   ...myself?

7) How would I want to do it differently next time?

8) Re-read your answers to the above questions. Reflect on what you have learned about how you contributed to the conflict you have dealt with. Be aware of how neither you nor the other person was to blame, but that you both had a point of view and feelings that would not allow you to hear each other objectively.

9) Now that you have explored feelings on both sides, experience the feeling of clarity and openness that comes from objective and open internal communication. This open communication with yourself leads to open and clear communication with others also. You can also use this exercise in many different situations to increase your awareness of how to communicate internally and externally.

HOW TO USE A JOURNAL TO IMPROVE YOUR INTERNAL COMMUNICATIONS

Writing in a special journal is another way for you to improve your internal process of communication. There are two ways in which the journal will work for you. *Getting in touch with your own inner imagery* is a way to uncover the deeper layers of your experience that are often crowded out by the noise of everyday concerns. Inner imagery comes when you put yourself in a meditative state and allow the mind to consciously relax. In all of the exercises below you will be able to record your imagery in your journal as you experience it in the moment. It is important to remember that imagery does not mean strictly "mental pictures." Imagery can also be feelings, sounds, situations or even smells that come into your inner awareness.

Holding an inner dialogue is another way for you to let the different parts of yourself become more conscious. The conversation actually takes the form of a written dialogue in which you become both speakers.

This dialogue technique is profoundly effective because you allow yourself to voice clearly both sides of any conflicting situation that arises in your life, where normally you might suppress one side or not even be aware it exists. You may find yourself saying things that you didn't even know you felt. You may encounter a surprising wisdom within you, that will move you towards a healing acceptance, understanding, and reconciliation of the opposing elements in the conflicts you experience.

A SUGGESTED WAY OF WORKING IN YOUR JOURNAL

1. *Keep a special daily record* of any situations that arise which seem to have a deeper emotional, mental or spiritual significance to you. It may be an interaction you have had with someone you work closely with, and you see something in your relationship you've never seen before. Note that experience, in a few words, in your daily record. You may have a deep experience in doing a new posture, or a breakthrough in your job. You may wake up with an unusual feeling about yourself. This daily record will give you material to work with when you want to get a perspective on your life by self-reflection in the form of journal writing.

2. *Schedule a time during the week* when you can review the events recorded in your daily record. Sit relaxed and ask yourself the question: "What does each of these events tell me about myself, about my emotions, about my physical body, about my mind and the way it works, about my spiritual growth?" Allow the important events to stand out in your awareness.

3. *Select one event or situation* in which your feelings seem unclear or unfinished. Sit with that situation for a moment, with your eyes closed. Enter into a meditative, quiet state. Allow all thoughts about it to dissolve, and simply feel the feelings that are involved in the situation. This is the stage in which your own inner images will rise to the surface spontaneously. Simply record these images as they come, without editing or judging them. After listing the images, re-read the list and ask, "What do these images tell me about myself?" The images are your own inner wisdom speaking to you in another language -- a language that is closer to your prana (that is, your feelings as you actually experience them, rather than as you merely think about them). Ask: "What are these images telling me about myself that I am not hearing in any other way?" Write down a brief statement about the situation, saying what you imagine the images are communicating about your own inner feelings, needs, thoughts, etc.

4. *You are now ready to enter into a dialogue with the situation.* In many conscious experiences you may feel the two different pulls on your energy, the pulls of conflicting feelings and of images you hold of yourself. Your conversation will take you

very deep into exploring these apparently conflicting elements within yourself when you concentrate on identifying the opposing messages you give yourself. In order to facilitate this process for the first few times, you may need to sit with your eyes closed to really get in touch with the feelings before writing. Some examples of arising conflicts that might be the two parties in your dialogue are:

- the weak you and the strong you.
- the successful you and the "failure" you.
- the you who wants to grow and the you who wants to live in the past or future.
- the closed, resistant part of you and the open, accepting part of you.
- your mind and your body.
- the fat you and the skinny you.
- the part of you that wants control and the part of you that wants to let go.
- the part of you that wants to be independent and alone, and the part of you that wants to be accepted by others.
- the part of you that wants to know who you are and the part of you that is afraid to know.
- the part of you that is feminine and the part of you that is masculine.
- the part of your job you like and the part of your job you don't enjoy.
- the part of you that feels vulnerable and resists change, and the part of you that is fearless and wants to try new experiences.

5. *Accept yourself as you are.* By allowing yourself the time to hear the conversations that constantly go on in your life, you have begun the process of accepting yourself honestly, as you are. As you accept, you open the door to understanding yourself and your needs. Your personal growth is the natural outcome of accepting, understanding and being ready to change the things you see in your life that hold you back from being yourself.

You can see that the list of possible conversations within yourself could go on endlessly. The above list will, at best, give a general idea of some areas where you might start to discover the people, experiences, feelings, fears, pleasures, and growths that make up the conscious events of your life. You will also discover that both of these two parts or sides of you are acceptable and natural -- that there is no need, in fact, to experience them as conflicting, but rather as complementary. Once you acknowledge them clearly, the need to negate one will drop away. They can both co-exist harmoniously, even if you must, of necessity, choose to act upon one only.

To hold an inner dialogue with yourself, go through the following steps:

a) Sit quietly for a moment and recall a situation

where you experienced some inner conflict or indecision. Identify what seem to be the two (or several) "voices" in the conflict, using the preceding list for guidance.

b) Start with one of those voices, and begin to hear what it is saying in the situation. As it becomes clear to you, begin to write down the words which express what it is saying. It is better not to think about it too much, as this may inhibit your experience; just allow the *feelings* to be expressed in words.

c) Now allow the other voice to respond to what the first voice said. Again let it come from your feelings without too much thinking. Let whatever words seem to express the feelings come, even if they seem strange to your rational mind, even if your first reaction is, "That isn't me; that isn't how I think!"

d) Allow the dialogue to continue, alternating the voices as long as it seems necessary for you to clarify the inner process that is going on. After a certain time, you will automatically feel "finished".

e) Go back over what you have written and see what you can learn from it.

f) Finally, turn to your higher self, your own inner guide and ask for guidance in interpreting and implementing what you have seen in yourself. This is best done through meditation; sitting quietly, relaxing consciously, and allowing the answers to flow to you spontaneously from that deep inner source of intuitive knowledge which becomes available to you at that time.

Every enlightened master describes our human nature as being both loving and able to receive love. Your true inner self is no different, so listening to yourself will provide you with the highest, most loving guidance possible.

Once we have clarified our own internal communication with ourselves, we are in a better position to begin to communicate clearly with others. Even then, of course, the way is full of pitfalls. There is an old saying: "There's many a slip 'twixt cut and lip", and there are many ways we can go astray even once we know what it is we want to communicate to the other. In this brief article, adapted from a lecture on communication given by Yogi Desai, are outlined seven key steps in communicating our feelings more clearly to other people.

There are two major prerequisites to clear communication with yourself and others. The first is self-responsibility: recognizing that you alone are the creator of all your life experiences; no one else causes you to feel what you feel. The second prerequisite is to see every difficulty that happens to you as a perfect opportunity for you to learn more about yourself and to grow in understanding, patience, tolerance and love. Then the aim of your communications will no longer be to change others, or to assign responsibility to them for creating difficulties, but simply to share yourself with them. If you can cultivate these two attitudes, all of your communication problems will begin to dissolve.

These guidelines will improve the quality of your communications. Each time you find yourself involved in any kind of miscommunication or misunderstanding, review these guidelines, using them as a checklist. They will help you to see where the miscommunication originated, how it has been perpetuated, and what you can do, in very specific ways, to right the situation. The more you work with them, the more you will internalize them until effortless communications begin to flow naturally through you.

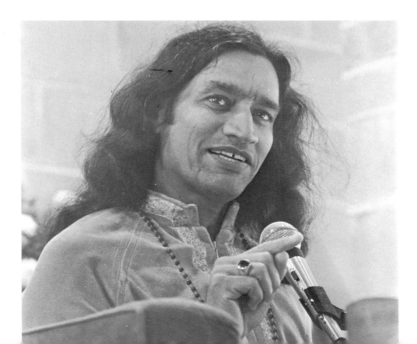

SEVEN STEPS TO CLEARER COMMUNICATION WITH OTHERS

by Yogi Amrit Desai

1. Examine the basic life attitudes which underlie your feelings. When you come to deeply understand that your happiness lies not in how others respond to you or how much you can change the world, but in changing the world inside of you, you will begin to change your perspective and your mind will become clear and objective. Those who have the greatest lack of objectivity are people who see the world as the source of their problems in miscommunication, and think that they themselves are always right. They are always trying to change other people and external conditions to solve their problems rather than working on themselves.

2. Accept responsibility for your own part in the misunderstanding. If you are involved in a misunderstanding with another person, stop and ask yourself the question, "Have I given enough time and understanding to the issue involved to ensure that I am fair and objective?" Then ask, "Have I chosen appropriate words and considerate language to communicate my feelings clearly?" If you learn only this much, you will create a unique capacity to express yourself honestly and clearly. Whether the other people understand or not is ultimately beyond your control. You can only help them so far. Communicating objectively with others, without blaming them, is of greatest importance.

3. Put yourself in the other's place. Open your heart. Ask yourself: "Am I being sensitive to how he/she is feeling right now? Is my heart open?" If you can be as attuned to the other person's feelings as you are to your own, you will be able to express what you are feeling in a sensitive way, and to choose the correct moment to express yourself. Even if you express what you feel with proper words, then clear communication will not result if you choose the wrong moment to say it. The right moment is when you are objective and open to admitting your own responsibility in the conflict. Only then can you explain to the other where the misunderstanding arose in a kind and loving manner, with carefully chosen words.

4. Become aware of what you want or expect from the other. Always ask, "What do I want from this person?" If you say what you imagine will make another person accept you, you will only be speaking the language of fear. What you want will invariably color both the words you choose and your body language. Miscommunication is frequently a clash between two people trying to guard their own security systems. If you understand what other people need for their own security and give them that, as a way of loving them, you will have conquered many miscommunication problems. Also, if you feel secure in communicating with other people then you create the same security for them.

5. Balance self-responsibility with patience and self-acceptance. As your consciousness begins to awaken and you develop a greater objectivity, you will be unable to place blame for your miscommunications totally on other people. You will see that you have more responsibility than you thought for your conflicts. You may even begin to place all the blame on yourself for the problems around you, and experience guilt, self-hatred, or an inferiority/superiority complex. It may even begin to seem that you have more problems than before your consciousness began to awaken. This is not so. You are simply more aware of what is happening. This is why accepting the responsibility for your communications needs to be balanced with self-acceptance, patience and self-love. As you see more, through your increased awareness, you will also begin to see your own needs for self-acceptance more clearly.

6. Develop a compassionate objectivity. When you develop objectivity you see the inside and outside of yourself *as you really are* without blame or guilt. This allows you to communicate with yourself -- to see where your problems really are. Compassionate objectivity is essential for moving from self-blame to self-acceptance. Then you can truly help others transcend their problems by offering them new perspectives that only loving objectivity allows. Psychological techniques may be able to bring people out of their difficulties, but they cannot give them the perspective that will sustain them long enough, in that condition, to transcend the problem. They will soon become the victims of similar problems again.

7. Recognize the ultimate benefit of good communication: realization of who you really are. With inner communication comes realization. You develop the capacity to become clear with yourself when you learn from experience that your problem lies within you and that, therefore, you are the only one who can remove it. A realization of this nature cannot come at a purely mental level. It can only happen experientially, at the heart level. You may hear certain things explained over and over again, but only when you have heard them experientially, through the heart, will you realize the implication of what is said and be able to practice it. You will be able to tell whether you have truly communicated with yourself by the change that each new realization brings to your life.

HOW TO MAKE YOUR SPEECH MORE POWERFUL

or: "I guess I'd really, sort of, like to, you know, learn to, er, speak, kind of, more clearly."

There are many small expressions and interjections in our everyday speech which weaken it and result in our not being understood clearly, or even well listened to by others. These little words have become so habitual that we are usually not aware of the frequency with which we use them. Even if we are aware, we may not realize the great effect they have, not only on how we communicate with others, but also on how others perceive us and how we perceive ourselves. Speech which is full of these words is either rather tedious to listen to or is so ineffectual that people actually do not hear what we are trying to say, or do not believe it.

We call these small words and phrases "qualifiers" and "nullifiers." They have come into existence in our speech at some time in the past when we felt insecure about what we were saying, or when we felt unable or unwilling, for some reason, to take full responsibility for our statements. Perhaps it started when we were young and we felt afraid that our feelings were not appropriate or would be criticized. Perhaps we were not sure of what we were saying, or not sure of the response we would get. These words then entered into our vocabulary and became habitual. The habits were then reinforced by the fact that other people had the same habit. There is a paradox here. Originally, we used these phrases out of insecurity. Now they are actually perpetuating our insecurity, because we sense that they are making our communication unclear. Our thoughts and words affect how we feel about ourselves, even if we are not always aware of this at the conscious level. Changing our speech patterns can have a profound effect on how we experience life.

As you read the following examples of unclear speech and the "corrected" versions that follow, say them aloud and be conscious of how you experience yourself differently. Then choose some examples of your own to practice with.

Qualifiers

These are the myriad little words we unconsciously interweave into our speech which have no real meaning or function in themselves. They may seem to have a purpose, but usually they simply attenuate our speech, making it weak and indecisive.

For example:

"*I guess* I *really* don't want to do what you suggest."
Substitute: "I prefer not to do what you suggest."

"It's *sort of* hard to say, *you know,* who is right."
Substitute: "I find it hard to say who is right."

"*Well,* I feel *kind of, you know...* upset."
Substitute: "Right now I'm feeling upset."

"It's *kind of* a touchy subject."
Substitute: "For me this is a difficult subject."

"I *just* want to let you know that..."
Substitute: "I want to let you know that..."

"*Maybe* [*perhaps*] we could talk about it some other time."
Substitute: "Could we please talk about it some other time?"

"It's *like* difficult to answer. *I mean...*"
Substitute: "I find that hard to answer."

Nullifiers

Nullifiers are words and phrases that tend to negate what we are saying or feeling, and to fix permanently in time our conception of ourselves and other people, removing all possibility of change. They are very subtle and insidious ways in which we prevent ourselves from owning our feelings and communicating clearly.

Again, as you read aloud both versions of the sentences below, notice how there is a subtle difference of feeling from one to the other.

1) Change *but* to *and.*

This admits the possibility of two parallel feelings existing in us at the same time, without any conflict or negation.

Example: "I really love you, but sometimes I get angry at you."
Instead say: "I really love you and..." etc.

2) Change *I know* to *I imagine.*

This gives the other person a chance to explain themselves and not feel judged or defined.

Example: "I know you're going to be angry with me."
Instead say: "I imagine you may be angry with me; of course I may be wrong."

3) Change *I can't* to *I prefer not to.* This owns responsibility for the attitude expressed, and thus gives us the power to change.

Example: "I can't talk to you right now."
Instead say: "I prefer not to talk to you right now."

4) Change *I have to* to *I choose to*

This is another opportunity to assume responsibility. It also avoids feeling resentment.

Example: "I have to go on a diet because I have high blood pressure."
Instead say: "I choose to go on a diet to regain my health."

5) Change *I should* to *I could.*

This again takes back responsibility from imaginary outside sources and "owns" the feeling.

Example: I should (ought to) get up early and go jogging."
Instead say: "I could get up early and go jogging." (Then choose to do it or not.)

6) Change *I don't know* to *I can find out.*

Instead of closing off all further possibilities, saying "I can find out" opens up new opportunities to grow, feel good, and help others.

Example: "I don't know what to do."
Instead say: "I can find out what to do."

7) Change *always/never* to an appropriate statement which is less restricted.

These two words are another example of limiting and permanently defining a person or a feeling. They can either be dropped altogether or replaced by sometimes, occasionally, until now, etc.

Example: "I always forget my wife's birthday."
Instead say: "I have forgotten my wife's birthday until now, but this time I will remember."

Example: "I never can get to a meeting on time."
Instead say: "Until now I haven't been able to get to a meeting on time. Now I can change."

In each case you will have observed that the second sentence feels more decisive, more clear and more direct. The speaker is really taking responsibility for what he or she is saying, without equivocation. In the first example of each sentence, the speaker is obviously ill at ease with what he or she is saying. They are like the politician who makes a statement, and then says quickly, "Don't quote me on that." When we use phrases like these qualifiers, we are indecisive. We want to say something yet, at the same time we don't want to because of the imagined consequences. Or more likely, we were at one time afraid; now we have more self-confidence, yet these words and phrases have become a deeply entrenched habit. Teenagers and young people in particular tend to use these qualifiers, because they are going through the insecurity of moving into the adult world where standards are different. Quite possibly we, too, picked up the habit at that time in our lives.

The solution, as we saw, is simply to drop these "extras" and say exactly what we feel. If we wish to soften our speech, it is better to do so by varying our tone of voice or simply by admitting that we are unsure of what we are about to say. There is no shame in saying: "I find it hard to express my feelings", "I'm not sure of what I am about to say," "I don't like to admit this because I feel vulnerable and weak", or "I don't like to be wrong, so I am afraid to say this."

Improving your communication skills will have a profound impact on your whole sense of well-being and progress towards Holistic Health. You will find yourself feeling consistently both more relaxed and more energetic, because your prana will be flowing more freely as a result of your ability to express yourself more freely. As you also learn to say what you want to say in a loving manner, you will feel more free in your interactions with others; you will feel confident in your ability to speak without hurting or antagonizing them. You will experience such a sense of satisfaction when you have managed to conduct, clearly, a communication that in the past would have left you feeling tense, frustrated, angry or depressed.

You will also experience others being more open to you, in a most surprising way, as they gain confidence in your openness and lack of desire to defend yourself or to manipulate them. Your ability and willingness to be real about your less noble feelings will open others' hearts to you, especially as you become able to express yourself with both honesty and gentleness.

True communication is more than just skill with words. It is the result of a gentle and open heart, which knows no other way to express itself than honestly and lovingly.

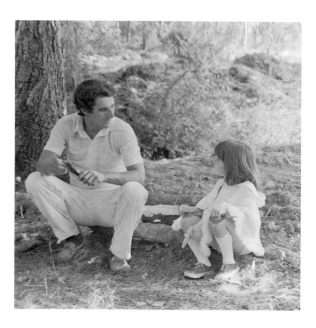

COMMUNICATION SKILLS II -- ACTIVE LISTENING

I Can't Hear You When You Talk While I'm Thinking about Myself

Another often neglected part of good communications is listening. We all value a good listener. We feel heard, understood, sympathized with, loved, when someone really listens to us without argument or judgment. Much of the therapeutic benefit of talking to a good listener, whether psychiatrist, clergyman or friend, is gained from the experience of being able to freely express what is bottled up inside without fear of the consequences. Very often, we cannot express our feelings to those closest to us, and about whom we feel what we feel, because we are afraid of the reactions. We fear hurt; we fear judgment; we fear criticism; we fear misunderstanding and mis-interpretation; we fear being rationalized out of our feelings; we fear being wrong; and, we fear, most of all, being overwhelmed and negated. So we either close up or seek an uninvolved and objective third party to whom we can "complain."

Yet, how often are we able to provide for others that open, non-judgmental listening ear that we, ourselves, appreciate and need so much? How often do we start out by "listening", only to jump in with our reactions, retorts, defenses and justifications? How often are we able to hear someone out, without comment, simply allowing them to express all that they are feeling? Even if we do remain silent, what is happening in our minds? Are we refuting them mentally, at every step, lining up our arguments in response? ("That's simply not true! That's so unfair. I can't let him get away with that.") Are we judging them mentally ("Oh, she always gets so emotional.")?

What seems to happen the most is that we are so busy reacting (there is so much noise of self-defensive thinking going on in our minds) that we simply cannot hear the other person properly. Even if we give the appearance of listening, our energies are all directed inwards to our own inner dialogues. And usually our eyes, if not our whole body language, reveal this. We've all experienced that feeling of "He/She's not with me -- not *really* listening." There's a glazed look in the eyes, a rest-lessness. Even if the person remains still, we sense in them a desire to move; we fear that, at any minute, they may look at their watch, spring to their feet, or interrupt us.

The true listener, in contrast, exudes a deep receptivity, a patience and endless willingness to be with us and let us express ourselves. Their eyes are like deep still pools, inviting us to plunge in. Their body language is saying "I am here for you as long as you need me. I am not here to refute you, to negate you, but simply to hear you, to receive you." Such people are truly rare. Even those who have made a profession of listening may not always have this quality; their listening sometimes has an air of abstraction, of practiced patience. Learning to truly listen is a sign of a willingness to love, or to learn to be more loving, for loving too is an art to be learned.

Knowing from experience what a great and loving gift true listening is, how can we learn to offer that gift to others? Some people may be born listeners, but most of us have to cultivate the art. The secret sounds deceptively simple (it's easy to understand, but hard to master): truly listening to others requires a certain degree of selflessness. It requires that we be able, for a period of time, to put aside our own needs and concerns and simply be a mirror for the other. In wordless empathy, we we allow others to see themselves more clearly, by hearing their own words and feelings, and putting aside our own personal responses. This is, for most of us, extremely hard to practice. We are so used to the responsive or reactive model where speakers alternate:

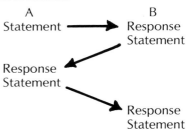

Communication, in this model, is like a tennis game -- and a very competitive one at that. Active listening, on the other hand, allows one player to keep on hitting, while the other simply receives the balls and lays them aside for a period of time.

Mastering the art of active listening is one of the most rewarding things in life that one can learn to do. Experiencing our own openness is a reward in itself; it feels wonderful to lay aside our own selfish concerns for a moment and just be there for the other person. The second reward is the depth and honesty of the other person's communication, which will be profound once they realize they can trust us, that our openness and patience are a gift of love and not a means of manipulation.

Listening to another, really listening, is the greatest gift of love that we can give.

HOW TO CULTIVATE THE ART OF ACTIVE LISTENING

Listening is at the heart of all communication, yet most of us listen only partially to each other. We then make assumptions or jump to conclusions which are not necessarily true because we haven't taken time to really hear the whole story. We call true listening "active listening" because it takes energy and it takes time. If you don't have either one, say so, and arrange to stop and listen when you have the necessary energy and time. Through really listening well, you come to learn more of who that other person really is; you allow them to feel understood and accepted by you; you hear your own self reflected in the other person; you help them to solve their own problems; you create an atmosphere of love and trust and set the stage for on-going communication between the two of you. You reduce their anxiety, allowing them to feel comfortable sharing with you; you create a friendship and love. Here is what you need to do:

1. Take time to really listen.

2. Sit in a relaxed, receptive way.

3. Establish and maintain eye contact.

4. Be on the same eye level (physical equality).

5. Remind yourself that the person is worthy of respect and attention (think of all the good things you know about them).

6. Drop your expectations and fears of what you're going to do.

7. Really hear the person.

8. Be here now (do not allow yourself to be distracted).

9. Be natural.

10. Be patient.

11. Try to feel the other person -- where is he or she? (Empathy means "to feel with.")

12. Drop your own responses, rationalizations, justifications, explanations, and just listen. Allow them to express their feelings without mental "buts" or verbal interjection. Hear them out.

Barriers to Active Listening

What can interfere with our ability to actively listen?

Many barriers can come up within our minds which interfere with our ability to really listen to another person; some of these we are conscious of and some we are not. Among those things preventing us from listening are:

1. Being distracted by something else.

2. Being overly worried about our own problems or concerns.

3. Fear of criticism from the other person.

4. Unfinished business (i.e., "I'm still reacting to what you did yesterday and I can't really hear what you're saying now.")

5. Second guessing (e.g. "I already know what you're going to say and so I have turned off my attention.")

6. Not being with the person (i.e., "I'm not seeing you but someone else you remind me of, so I hear his voice instead, not yours.")

ACTIVE LISTENING MEANS TRUE ACCEPTANCE OF THE OTHER PERSON...EXACTLY AS HE OR SHE IS.

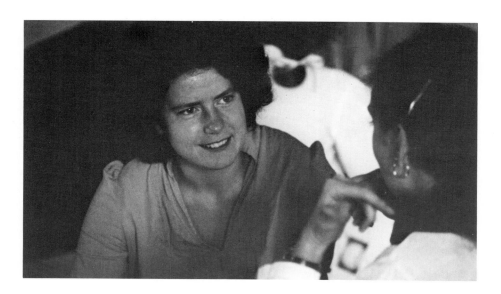

BEYOND CLEAR COMMUNICATION

The next step after learning to communicate clearly is to learn to communicate lovingly. Once we know clearly what it is we feel, we need to learn to find words which express that feeling in a way that is both honest and loving. It is good to recognize that we are angry, it is not so good to express that anger by shouting or speaking in a hostile way to the person who is the target of our anger, because it will make it harder for clear and loving communication to happen between us.

The following is a series of pointers excerpted from the teachings of Yogi Desai on how to see your communications with others as a way to love them more.

COMMUNICATION THROUGH LOVE

by Yogi Amrit Desai

Failure to communicate is not verbal inability so much as lack of attunement to the other, lack of love for the other. Love communicates better than words because the feeling is transmitted directly. No matter how good the words, without love the message will not get across. The other person will be deaf to your logic, even to the truth, until you add a little love. Instead of trying to explain, try to love.

• Learning how to communicate clearly is a gift, not only to yourself but to others. By helping others to understand you, you are opening them up to you and to the rest of life. You are providing them with new ears, enabling them to really hear and understand you. Your inability to communicate does not merely result in your not getting the message across to others. You are closing them down, shutting off their experience of you, simply by not being able to choose the right words. You may even create enemies for yourself, though your intentions were good, if you don't know the right language. Learning how to communicate well is thus a first step to learning how to love unconditionally.

• One very deeply-rooted principle in human nature is the craving to be appreciated. If you can fulfill that craving in someone else, then you have really communicated. Of course this should only be done with the highest motive -- the pure selfless desire to help others and to extend love to them.

• If you can be really unattached in your communication, if your motive is pure and selfless, then you will have no difficulty being heard, because what you want from that person, if it is based on unconditional love and understanding, is the same as what his own higher nature would want him to do. Appeal to the higher instincts in the other, and you will draw out the highest response in that person.

• If you speak softly, gently and truthfully, then you are developing a silent strength in your language; it will have the ring of truth when you speak. If you watch your thoughts, taking care to only harbor kind, loving and truthful thoughts, they too will have a power. People who are in the habit of lying and being dishonest have very confused minds. They're always restless, tense and fearful, and no one pays much attention to what they say.

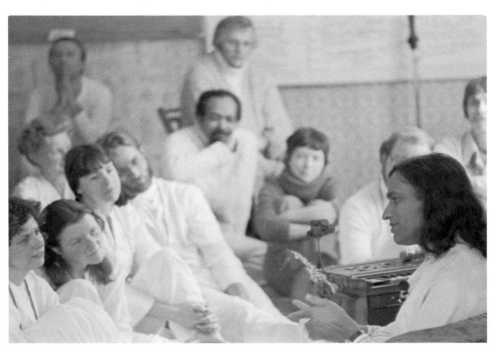

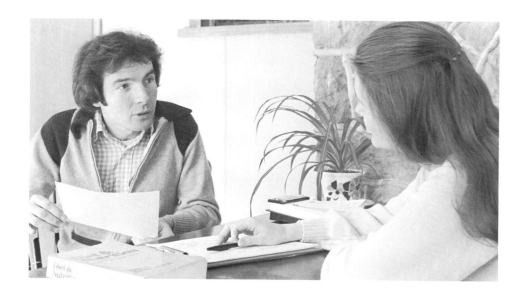

• It is important to be accurate and specific when you speak. To generalize and exaggerate is very harmful to your consciousness because your subconscious mind is not discriminating; it takes everything you say quite literally.

Always speak and think positively about other people. This gives them the freedom to change. If you criticize and condemn others, you are reinforcing their weakness and giving it deeper roots. If you find this difficult, it is because you, yourself, don't want to change. If you are willing to grow, to be flexible, you will allow that to others, too.

• Be economical in your speech. Only say what is necessary, and avoid wasting energy in unnecessary emotional expressions. When you use your energy in a wrong way, it always rebounds on you.

• When you experience negative or unpleasant emotions, the most important thing is to recognize that it is natural and normal to feel that way. You have every right to experience what you are feeling, but you don't have a right to impose it on others. So, you must take care to explain to them, in a courteous way, that you are experiencing a negative emotion that is clouding your ability to communicate with them. If you tell them that you are experiencing that, but you don't want to project it onto them, they will accept it. But if you impose your anger on others, you will simply receive anger in return. If you are able to express your negative feelings positively and objectively, then you will reap positive benefits for yourself.

• All negative emotions (anger, hatred, jealousy) come from one source: you wanted something from that person and you didn't get it. The more specifications you have about how life should be, the more occasion you will have to get angry.

• Do not try and get sympathy from others for your problems. Sympathy will make you feel justified, and then you will not take responsibility for your own emotion; you will not grow. Accept your negative feelings without spreading them, knowing that they will not last. They will pass by. They are a part of life and growth, just as storms are a part of life.

• The next step after accepting your negative emotions is to understand them, to find out where they come from and to see clearly what part your own selfish interest plays in them. Then you can be completely objective about them. Your negative feelings will dissolve -- they are only the result of your misunderstanding. When you are afraid to do this, you lose your capacity to be objective; you don't even want to face the fear. You are afraid of the fear and this doubles it. If you face the fear fairly and squarely, once and for all, instead of avoiding or ignoring it, it will never come back to haunt you.

• Remember that just as you are trying to grow, so is everyone else, in his or her own way. It may not be your way. It may not even be apparent at all. But there is an inner evolutionary urge in all of us. So, remember the prayer of St. Francis: instead of wanting to be understood, try to understand the other person and say, "You're doing it your way, and that's fine." You will never get complete understanding from others anyway, because no one can understand you the way you understand yourself. But you do have it in your power to understand others, to accept them as they are, and to love them.

• When love exists, communication of the highest order occurs spontaneously. This communication is really a communion. It flows from heart to heart rather than from head to head. This is true communication.

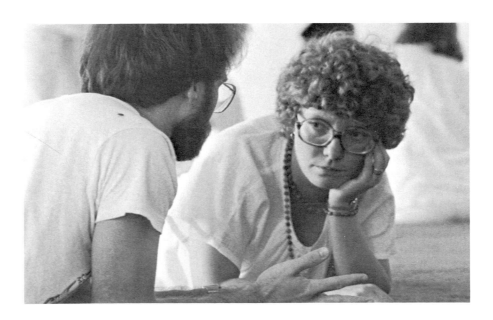

HOW TO EXPRESS FEELINGS AND GIVE FEEDBACK

For many of us, expressing feelings is much harder than expressing opinions, facts or theories. If you listen to people's conversations, you will notice that very often they are either describing things, events and people (books, movies, politics, friends) or else exchanging facts and opinions about these topics. Very rarely are these conversations about personal feelings. The reason is that talking about feelings involves a risk. Expressing our feelings is revealing who we really are. If the other person does not like who we are, we may find it difficult to like and accept ourselves. It seems to be particularly risky if the feelings we have are those commonly labelled "negative", "weak", or "unacceptable" such as anger, frustration, or hurt. And for some people it is simply not considered appropriate to discuss feelings at all.

Part of the reason that we are reluctant to express our feelings to others is that we do not feel confident of our ability to say what we feel in a way that is both honest and, at the same time, loving and kind. Experience has taught us that if we do not succeed in finding the correct words and tone of voice to give feedback about our feelings, then we may provoke anger, hostility or hurt in the other person. Out of fear of the imagined consequences, we often remain silent even when we feel it would be useful to give feedback. As a result, we bottle up feelings and then may harbor resentment against others, or lose our tempers later and express those feelings in a way which does, in fact, provoke the very reaction we originally feared.

Giving feedback and expressing our feelings can be an easy and rewarding experience if we learn a few simple guidelines and a slightly new point of view about our feelings. The result of being able to give feedback lovingly and clearly is a tremendous sense of release and freedom, and also a new openness between ourselves and others; a new and often unforeseen liking and respect, instead of distance and anxiety.

Here are some guidelines for giving feedback, structured in the Three A's format.

Awareness

1. *Become aware of what you are feeling.* It is very important to clearly *recognize the feeling* that you wish to share with another. Simply knowing that you feel "upset" or "uncomfortable" will not enable you to become really clear about the nature of your feelings. You will need to refine your awareness until you can be more precise and say to yourself, "I feel hurt, appreciated, unloved, loved, unconsidered, afraid, confident, angry," etc.

2. *Understand the true origin of your feelings.* Often we make the mistake of believing that we are experiencing a certain feeling because someone else did something and "made" us feel that way. In fact, we are the creators of our own feelings and experiences. It is our own *interpretation* of the other person's acts or words that makes us feel the way we do, not the acts themselves. The idea that we alone are responsible for our feelings is a hard one for many of us to process. Yet we need to be able to accept it fully and wholeheartedly if we are to go on to express our feelings and feedback objectively and lovingly. It is only our past conditioning that makes us believe that we experience hurt, anger or pain because of

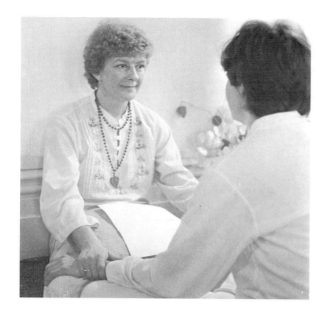

someone else's actions. Once we can take back the responsibility for all that we are feeling it gives us a tremendous power and control over our own lives. We no longer have to feel like a victim or a bystander; we are no longer giving to others the power to decide how we will experience our lives. Other people too will be more open to us once they see that we no longer have a desire to blame them for what we are feeling, and they will be more willing to assume responsibility for their own actions. So ask yourself:

a)What do I believe or imagine that the other person is telling me through their words and actions?

b) How is my feeling a result of this belief?

In actual fact, the other person may not have meant what you imagined, and so you may have a pleasant surprise when you check it out with them.

3. *Examine your motivation for sharing your feelings.* Once you are clear on the first two points, you can go on to the third one, which is to know clearly *why* you want to share what you want to share. If your motivation to share is not objective, you will find that your feedback is not as well received as you would like. We often tell ourselves that we simply want to let the other person know how we are feeling, when in fact, deep down, we really want them to change their behavior so that it is more acceptable to us, or to make them feel responsible, or even guilty, for the way they have "made" us feel. This is a perfectly understandable and human reaction. We may not recognize it because we think it is "bad" and therefore we believe we should not feel this way. However, once we see and accept this motivation, we are freed to go on to the next step, which is to

find a more loving and objective reason for sharing our feelings. Some positive reasons for giving feedback might be:

a) to simply learn whether the other person meant what you imagined they meant.

b)to clarify a miscommunication or situation so that it will not occur again.

c) to fearlessly and openly reveal yourself to the other person, *as you are,* so that they know you better and are able also to be more open with you.

d) to provide them with objective information on their environment so that they can decide whether or not they wish to modify their words or behavior in order to interact more harmoniously with others. (You will have to be open here to the possibility that they may choose *not* to change, and to feel OK with that. That is their right.)

Acceptance

1. *Accepting full responsibility for creating your own feelings* -- what past programing is causing you to react in the way you do -- then you will gradually be able to come to a point of complete acceptance of responsibility. You will also begin to feel very free.

2. *Accept the other person's response to your feedback.* It may be that no matter how objective and loving your feedback is, the other person is still not able to be open to you. This is because they too have their own internal "agenda"; their own misconceptions about what you are saying and why, based on their past conditioning. Your ability to accept their reaction to your feedback with equanimity is a test of your original objectivity. If you feel frustrated, hurt, or angry, then ask yourself: "What was it I wanted from the exchange? How did I expect or want them to respond?" In this way, giving feedback is a means of learning more about yourself as well as giving the other person the opportunity to learn more about you and about themselves.

Feedback involves taking risks: the risk of learning something about yourself that you didn't know before (and that you may not at first like) and the risk of being misunderstood or not accepted. Yet these are worthwhile risks, because you also stand to gain a new love, understanding and respect from others for your fearlessness and your realness.

Adjustment

Now you are ready to give your feedback, but before you do, check it against the list of criteria that follows, to ensure that it meets all the requirements for objective and loving communication. As you do this ongoingly, you will

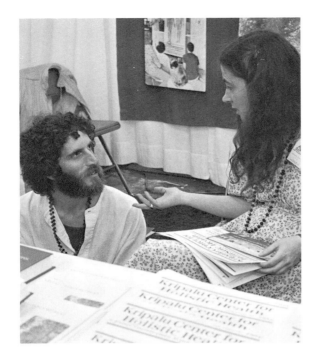

experience a growing confidence in your ability to express your feelings clearly to others.

Loving and Objective Feedback is:

1. ASKED FOR, OR AGREED TO, WILLINGLY

Feedback is most helpful and openly received when it has been asked for. If not, then at least ask the person whether or not they are willing to hear you.

FOR EXAMPLE:

Feedback imposed: "I need to share something with you right now."

Agreed to: "I have some feelings that I think would be helpful for me to share with you. Would you be willing to listen to them? When would be a good time?"

2. WELL-TIMED

Although feedback is most helpful right after the situation has occurred, other factors must be considered. Is the situation appropriate? Is the other person ready and willing to hear it at that time?

FOR EXAMPLE:

Ill-timed: "I just have to tell you right now that I got really angry at you this morning when...oh dear! I didn't realize you had a hard time with your boss at the office today. I didn't mean to upset you. "

Well-timed: "I'm glad I waited to share this with you. I feel more comfortable knowing you are rested and relaxed."

3. OWNS RESPONSIBILITY

As discussed above, blaming others only results in them feeling defensive and closed to you. It is more helpful to use statements which clearly show that you accept that your feelings are a result of your interpretations of the other's actions.

FOR EXAMPLE:

Blaming the other: "You make me so angry when you come home late for supper."

Accepting responsibility: "When you come home late for supper, I imagine that you don't care about my feelings, and as a result of imagining this, I get upset."

Tips: To help you in remaining with your own responsibility, use statements beginning with "I" as much as possible rather than "you", "it", etc. For example:

Instead of "It makes me mad..." say *"I get mad..."*
Instead of "You really have to laugh when..." say *"I really have to laugh when..."*
Instead of "One can't help being upset when..." say *"I become upset when..."*
Instead of "We all make mistakes" say *"I make mistakes."*
Instead of "People do the silliest things" say *"I do the silliest things."*

Notice how you feel differently when you make the statement the second way. You are really "owning" the feelings involved rather than making them general statements about life which are intellectual rather than experiential.

CHECK OUT THE OTHER'S FEELINGS AND INTENTIONS

Ask questions which verify where the other person was coming from when they spoke/acted, rather than making statements ascribing motives to them which may be totally inaccurate.

FOR EXAMPLE:

Doesn't check out others' feelings: "I wish you wouldn't be so impatient with me."

Checks out: "When you spoke to me just now I imagined you were feeling impatient with me. Were you feeling impatient, or was something else happening?"

5. IS DESCRIPTIVE RATHER THAN EVALUATIVE

By simply describing your own feelings without placing a value judgment on the actions/words of the other person it leaves them free to respond without defensiveness or rationalization.

FOR EXAMPLE:

Evaluative: "It is so inconsiderate of you to always keep me waiting when we are going somewhere."

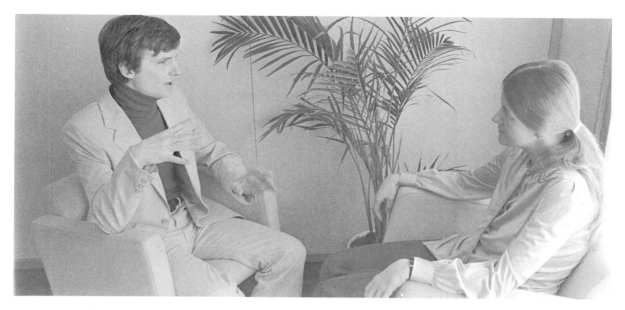

Descriptive: "It seems to me that you are often late when we are going somewhere, and I must admit I don't like to have to wait. as I'm not a patient person. Can we work this out together?"

6. IS SPECIFIC RATHER THAN GENERAL.

This helps the other person not to feel they are always "in the wrong" and shows them it is not them as a person you are unhappy with, but simply a single aspect of their behavior.

FOR EXAMPLE:

General: "You always try to dominate the situation."

Specific: "Just now, when you said that, I imagined that you did not want to listen to what I had to say, and I felt unhappy."

7. TAKES ACCOUNT OF THE RECEIVER'S NEEDS ALSO

The receiver of your feedback will be more open to your feelings if you show that you are open to their needs too.

FOR EXAMPLE:

Takes account of the speaker's needs only: "I don't like it when you wake me up early in the morning. It's not fair."

Takes receiver's needs into account also: "I don't like it when you wake me up early, yet I do understand your need to get up at that time. Can we work out a compromise?"

8. IS CHECKED AFTERWARDS

There are two good reasons for checking back to see how your communication was received. First, you ensure that the other person has really understood what you wanted them to understand, and second, you find out how they are feeling about what you have shared -- you get feedback on your feedback!

FOR EXAMPLE:

Unverified communication: "Well, that's all I wanted to say; thanks for listening."

Verified: "Please tell me what you heard me say, so that I can be sure I communicated clearly. How do you feel about what we have just shared?"

9. IS DIRECTED TOWARD BEHAVIOR THE RECEIVER CAN DO SOMETHING ABOUT IF THEY CHOOSE TO.

This avoids generating a feeling of frustration or even despair in the receiver.

FOR EXAMPLE:

Directed at something unchangeable/irrational: "The way you talk to me makes me unhappy because it reminds me of my mother. She always talked like that."

Directed at changeable behavior: "When you spoke to me just now, in a way that seemed rather abrupt to me, I felt threatened. I realize this is just an old habit pattern, because it reminded me of the way my mother sometimes spoke. As a child I felt anxious, because I didn't realize she was just tired. I thought she didn't love me. I wanted to tell you this so that you will understand my reactions better."

These examples will give you a feel for ways to take more responsibility for your feelings so that others will be comfortable and unthreatened when you share with them. You will begin to find that others will welcome your feedback, because they get to know you better and to trust your objectivity. Often it comes as a great relief to know for sure how the other person is feeling; it may not be nearly as bad as what we are imagining! Also, you will come to feel really good about yourself as your capacity to be more 'real' with others increases. Try it and see!

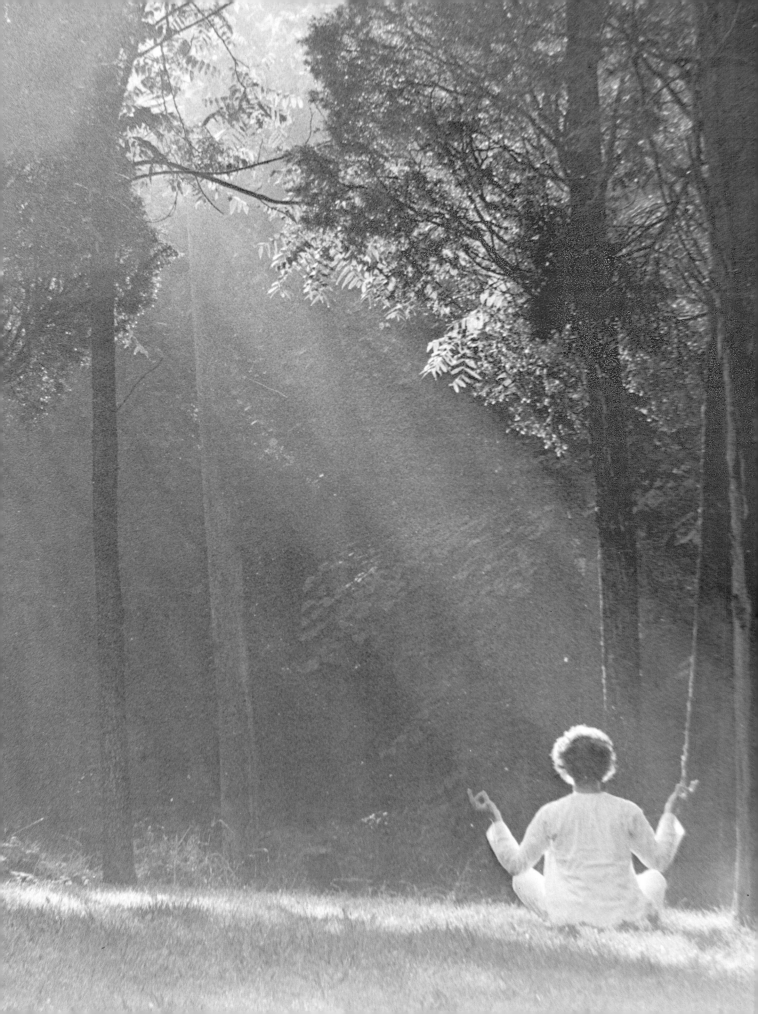

WAY SEVEN
meditation and spiritual attunement

SPIRITUAL ATTUNEMENT?

The words may not be familiar; the experience is. You have experienced many moments of spiritual attunement throughout your life. These moments have come to you in varying ways, depending on your temperament, your lifestyle, your beliefs. Perhaps there was a moment when you felt completely at peace with the world, when everything seemed to be unfolding as it should. Your every need seemed to be met at that moment; your every desire stilled or fulfilled. You may have experienced it in those timeless moments of ecstasy and joy at the beauties of nature, as you walked in the mountains or by the ocean at sunset. Perhaps it has been more of a calm sensation of warmth, fulfillment and gratitude, as you sat in gentle communion with the ones you love. Maybe it has come to you as a feeling of profound satisfaction and absorption as you completed a work of art or even a simple craft, and gloried in your own creative energies. It may have come to you in a place of worship or in private prayer. There are as many ways to experience spiritual attunement as there are people in this world. Yet what the experiences all have in common seems to be their evanescent quality. They are of limited duration. Afterwards, we are again plunged in the workaday world with all its excitements and difficulties.

Yet this need not be the case. Spiritual attunement, like anything else, can be cultivated. We can, with practice, learn to make this deeply satisfying and joyful feeling a part of our everyday experience. Peace, joy and satisfaction are our natural birthright as human beings, not special blessings conferred on us very occasionally. They need not come to us out of the blue, completely by chance. We have lost the art of experiencing spiritual attunement ongoingly because we have not believed in it as our inalienable birthright. We have somehow come to believe that such moments are rare, unpredictable and uncontrollable.

All we have to do to experience contentment, joy and peace more often is to open ourselves to the possibility of it, and to believe it is attainable and that we deserve to experience it. Then we can begin to find ways to bring it into our lives ongoingly.

What is spiritual attunement? The basic ingredient seems to be a feeling of completeness, of oneness, of unity. Oneness between oneself and the universe, and between all aspects of oneself. If oneness is not always the conscious ingredient, then at least there is absence of conflict, and absence of disease. The experiences of the body, the thoughts of the mind and the aspirations of the spirit (the higher self) are all in harmony. How can we work consciously to bring that harmony into our lives more often? What do we need to do?

Your Body -- Your Instrument

Imagine for a moment that you are a violinist, about to take your seat with the orchestra to play a symphony. How will you prepare yourself? First, you have to ensure that all the strings of your instrument are at the correct tension or the sounds they make will be simply noise or dull twanging.

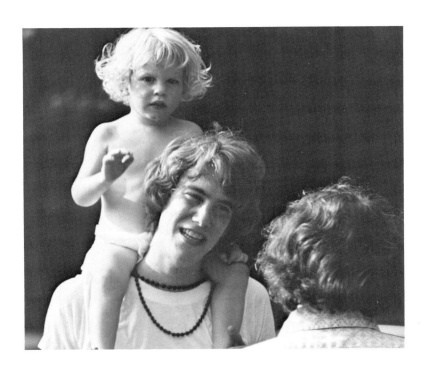

Each separate string has to be tuned to its appropriate pitch. Then the strings have to be attuned to each other. However beautiful each string sounds when played alone, if it is not attuned to the other three the result will still not be music and harmony, but discord and stridency. And even when this is accomplished and you take your seat with the orchestra, you will still have to attune your instrument to the instruments of those with whom you are about to play, or again, the result will not be harmony. There will be no symphony. This group attunement is attained by each instrument being tuned to one standard, universal pitch.

Now see the violin as a symbol for the human being. The human instrument has three strings: body, mind and spirit. Each needs to be perfectly tuned within itself first. The body has to be perfectly healthy and the mind clear and objective. The spirit must be pure and free (which it always has been from the beginning; it just needs to be recognized). Then these three have to be attuned to each other. One string always has to serve as the basis, the ground against which all the others are tuned. In the human being this ground is the spirit -- our indwelling prana in its most subtle manifestation. Once we have attuned our body and mind to our prana, through the many methods suggested in this book, we will find that we are unerringly attuned to all that surrounds us, for we are in harmony with the pitch of nature itself, with the vibration of the universe. Our own prana always resonates in harmony with the universal prana.

The key to all health, peace and happiness is learning how to be finely attuned to our prana, in body and mind, at every moment of the day.

There are two levels on which we can work to bring about the alignment of body and mind with the needs of the spirit. The first is through practice of specific techniques, and the second is through further heightening of our daily awareness of the voice of prana.

The material that follows explains the use of meditation as a tool for pranic spiritual awareness, along with an article by Yogi Desai about a unique way to be aware of our thoughts and movements in daily life, so that life itself becomes an expression of spirit. First, however, complete the Self-Discovery Experience which follows.

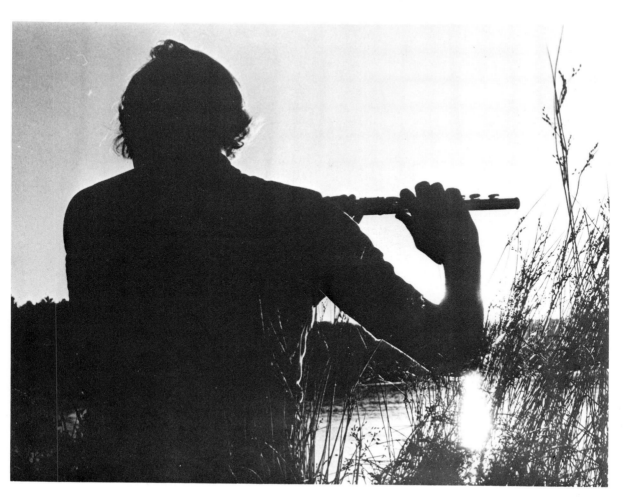

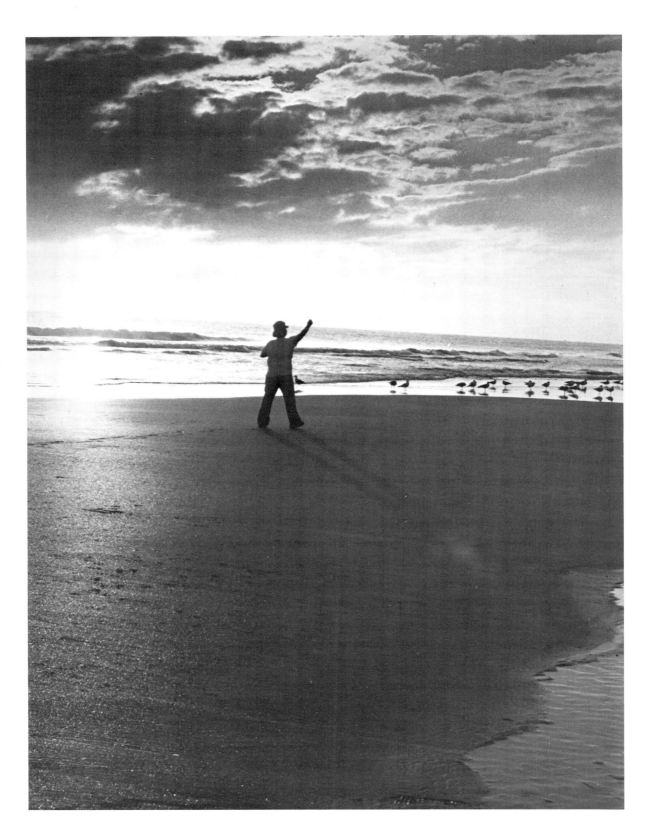

Self-Discovery Experience 14

Attuning To Your Higher Self

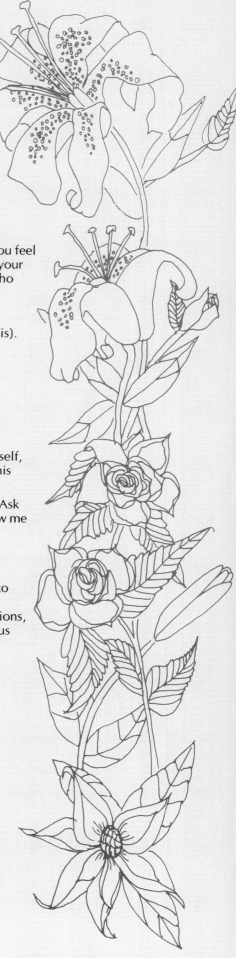

Awareness

1. Take an inner inventory. List all of the times, plans, circumstances in which you feel truly "in tune" with your true inner Self. List them freely. Close your eyes and let your mind acknowledge even the briefest and most subtle moments of being close to who you really are.

2. Arrange these in order of *frequency* of occurence. List the "top ten".

3. Arrange your original list in order of *potency* (i.e. how powerful the experience is). List the top five.

4. Now examine the top five of each list. Are they the same or different?

Acceptance

1. Look at how often or seldom you are in the position to experience the five most potent circumstances that leave you fully in touch with yourself.

2. Examine one that you would like to feel more often. Explore tendencies in yourself, in your habits, in your attitudes that affect how often you practice or experience this form of attunement.

3. Attune to your inner wisdom and give yourself some compassionate guidance. Ask your higher self: "How should I go about attuning myself more to your needs? Show me where I am neglecting you, and how I can reflect you more."

Adjustment

Reflect on the guidance. Discover ways to practically implement it. Don't forget to consider how friends or loved ones might be able to assist you, especially if you sincerely share your aspiration with them. Give them the opportunity to ask questions, as they may not understand right away. Try to be flexible and achieve a harmonious integration of their needs and your own.

MEDITATION AND THE SEARCH FOR PEACE OF MIND   *by Yogi Amrit Desai*

Getting "Enough"

We are all, in our different ways, searching for lasting peace of mind. Few people are fortunate enough to find it. Many things block the way to true inner peace. The first impediment is the belief that peace of mind depends on external, material security. People say: "I want to live in peace and enjoy life, but I must have security for that. I must have enough security to provide adequately for myself and my family."

What do these words "enough" and "adequate" really mean? How much is enough? How will you know when you have enough external security? Is it when it gives you complete peace of mind? If so, you will never get enough. It will never give you the peace of mind you seek, because external, material security and success alone are not capable of providing you with true, lasting peace of mind.

Look around you. There are so many people who still do not have peace of mind even after highly successful lives and great material security. For years these people have looked forward to retirement, to having enough material success to experience freedom from worry. They dreamed that when they retired, they would have enough time and resources to really enjoy life. But when the time comes, and they have all the luxury, material resources and time to enjoy life to the fullest, what happens? The cherished dream turns into a nightmare for many of them. Their freedom becomes the worst form of punishment. They are totally unable to enjoy it because they do not possess the missing ingredient -- peace of mind.

Security - or Serenity

Such people are so restless that they are completely unable to enjoy a relaxed life. They have developed an unbreakable habit of needing activity, of needing problems to solve and things to do all day long. Their search for security, which started out as a means to an end, became the end in itself. The harder they strained their physical, emotional and mental resources to attain the elusive goal of security, the more impossible it became for them to withdraw from their activities and enjoy the peace which these very activities were supposed to bring. They became so preoccupied with their search for "enough" success and security that, without realizing it, they sacrificed both their health and their peace of mind. Now that they have enough material security, they have neither the physical health nor the mental peace to enjoy it. They have traded serenity for security. It is a poor exchange.

The search for peace of mind through the acquisition of material security is an illusion. The restless seeking and striving that this search requires becomes a habit too strong for most people to break. The tension seriously impairs their health. Such a life is like that of a mouse running on a treadmill. There is no freedom. The only choice you have is to run faster or slower. The faster you run, the more you are blind to what is happening around and within you. And there is no point of arrival -- ever.

Peace of Mind, Now

This does not mean that you should give up all concern for material security for yourself and your family. Not at all. Simply recognize that external security will never bring you the lasting peace of mind that you seek. Ask yourself "What is the true meaning of security to me? Is it simply external success and material prosperity? Or does it also concern my state of mind? My physical health? My emotional well-being? Is it for the future, or is it for now as well?" When you have the answers to these questions, ask one more: "Do I need to change my life, or my attitude, to provide myself with the peace of mind I seek -- right now?"

Peace of mind, like restlessness and dissatisfaction, is a habit. It is either nurtured or destroyed by how you live each day, each moment, of your life. It comes from within you, not from external objects or events. Because it is an attitude, it can be cultivated. Because it is a habit, it can be acquired through constant repetition and practice. Meditation is one of the most powerful tools available to human beings in their search for lasting peace of mind. Meditation helps on two levels. First, it helps you to go within and find, in the peaceful depths of your being, the answers to all your questions and searching. Second, it brings balance and clarity to your mind and strength to your will. These qualities enable you to transform your old habits of restlessness and tension into new patterns of health-giving peace and self-fulfillment.

The Searching Mind

Meditation works in the following way. The mind is, by its very nature, restless and searching. It is searching for pleasure and satisfaction. This it hopes to find from two sources: external objects, events and people, and internal memories of objects, events and people.

The mind automatically divides all experiences into two categories: pleasurable and unpleasurable. It then seeks out pleasurable experiences and memories, and tries to avoid the unpleasurable ones. The stronger these likes and dislikes are, the more the mind is restless and overactive.

Strong likes and dislikes generate strong emotions. The stronger the emotions, the greater the energy they consume. Strong emotions are blinding. They prevent the mind from seeing truth objectively and making the right decisions. A mind that is swayed by strong likes and dislikes is unable to find a solution to even the easiest of problems; its confusion complicates the simplest situations. We have all experienced this at some time. Even the wisest people are capable of acting foolishly when their minds are swayed by conflicting emotions, desires or fears. They have no access to their store of wisdom when their minds are restless and unsettled.

Meditation calms and focuses the restless mind. A steady, calm mind opens the door to all wisdom and knowledge because prana can flow freely through it, just as prana flows more freely through a relaxed body. Prana is the universal life force, the universal Mind, the source of all wisdom and knowledge. A restless mind is a veil between us and this universal source of knowledge. As soon as the mind is calmed and emptied of conflicting thoughts and desires, true wisdom and knowledge begin to flow into the space created. This emptying is the source of all creativity, all intuition, all wisdom. As your mind becomes calm and still, and you enter into the depths of your being, you will contact this universal intelligence in your heart as an experience of peace and love.

Emptying the Mind to Receive Wisdom

Meditation is the process of emptying the mind so that it can receive this universal wisdom, peace and love, which paradoxically is already there, deep within you, waiting to be contacted. In meditation you begin to dissolve your restlessness, your intense likes and dislikes, your attachments and your fears. You no longer see life in terms of opposites to be sought or avoided. Ultimately, when it is mastered, meditation becomes a spontaneously-experienced state of thought-free stillness and ecstasy. But in order to reach that very high level, specific techniques must be practiced to tame the restless mind, which has had a lifetime of unfettered activity.

All meditation techniques have one common goal: to help meditators achieve the stillness of mind that will allow them to make deep contact with their own inner source of wisdom, peace and fulfillment. Beginning meditation techniques are more properly called concentration techniques. Concentration techniques focus the thoughts, which are normally scattered into many different directions. This scattering diffuses the energy of the mind and causes tension and restlessness. Concentration focuses the scattered energy. Focused energy leads to the experience of inner peace and calm. This form of concentration-

meditation is described in the following way by the great yogi Patanjali in about the 4th century B.C.: "Meditation occurs when all thoughts begin to flow in an unbroken chain towards one subject, without interruption from thoughts of unrelated subjects."

Concentration, as such, can be on any subject, mundane or spiritual. Whatever the subject, the mind will be trained to focus its energies on a single thing. Meditation, on the other hand, focuses on subjects which are spiritually inspiring. Its purpose is to awaken the meditator to higher states of awareness and spiritual consciousness.

Kripalu Yoga Meditation-in-Motion

There are many different types and techniques of meditation. Each one is suitable to a certain temperament and level of spiritual development. Classical seated meditation, known as Raja Yoga, is usually practiced after a certain level of physical skill in Hatha Yoga postures has been attained. Kripalu Yoga is different from both of these practices, yet combines the benefits of both. It also eliminates the drawbacks they sometimes hold for Westerners. It has been my privilege to originate and develop Kripalu Yoga as a technique especially suited to the Western temperament,

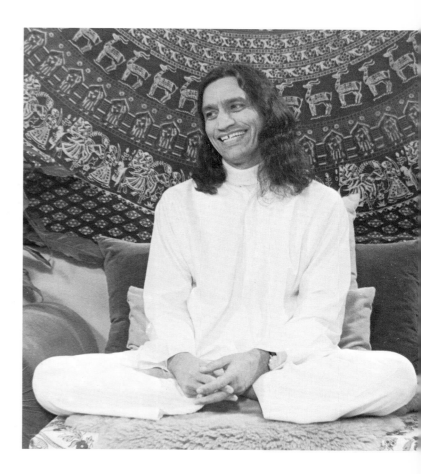

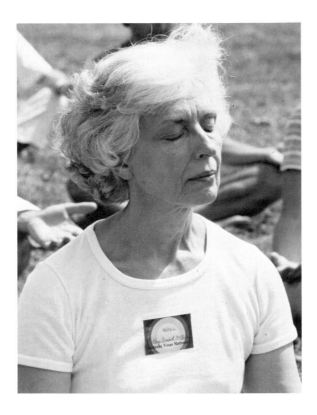

which is highly active, both physically and mentally. When many Westerners practice seated Raja Yoga meditation, their bodies become restless after a while and this is a distraction from meditation. On the other hand, when they are practicing Hatha Yoga, they are often not taught to concentrate their minds sufficiently on the postures, with the result that their thoughts roam restlessly and they do not gain full benefit from the exercises. In both cases peace of mind and a deeply meditative state are elusive.

In Kripalu Yoga, the body movements themselves are the focus of concentration. Through specific ways of moving and breathing (see Way Two: Kripalu Yoga) a powerful magnetic field is created which keeps the mind totally concentrated on the movements being performed. A deeply meditative state results -- one that is attained almost effortlessly. Kripalu Yoga leads you in five stages from the level of simple concentration to the transcendent stage where both meditation and movement are spontaneous. At this level you will experience an intense awareness of the divine nature of prana and a deep sense of inner peace, contentment and fulfillment.

Holistic Meditation

The regular practice of meditation will bring profound and far-reaching benefits to your life, no matter what your age or background. You will first begin to experience a level of physical relaxation and inner peace that you have never known before, a peace which continues long after the period of actual meditation is over. Your mind will become clearer, more focused, more powerful, enabling you to make decisions and take action with greater ease than ever before. Your creativity and intuitive powers will be awakened. You will find yourself gaining the ability to remain calm even in the midst of stressful and conflicting situations. As a result of this increased calmness you will experience a greater ability to accept things as they are. You will find that you also accept other people, and yourself, as they are too. Your interpersonal relationships will thus become more successful and harmonious.

All these benefits will come from the regular practice of short periods of meditation. Kripalu Yoga's Meditation-in-Motion is the ideal form of meditation for those interested in Holistic Health, because it works with the whole person -- body, mind and spirit. It is holistic meditation.

Three Simple Meditation Techniques

Three meditation techniques are described here. The first, and simplest, will give you a feel for the basic elements of meditation. You can then apply these basics as you experiment with the other two. Remember, however, that the key to progress in meditation is to pick one technique and practice it regularly, rather than skipping from technique to technique.

Preparation

In each case, the prerequisites are the same:

1. Choose a quiet, secluded place where you will not be interrupted or disturbed (but if a disturbance comes up, do not be disturbed at being disturbed!)

2. Choose a time when you can do it each day at that hour, so that you become "conditioned", in a positive sense. Your mind and body will be trained to become quieter and more introspective at that time.

3. Dim the lights and, if you like, light candles and/or incense to create a conducive environment.

4. If you can wash, shower or bathe beforehand you will feel much more receptive.

5. Wearing clean clothes (some meditators choose white clothing) can also help to create a vibration of "specialness", of calm and peace, of being lifted out of the usual hurly-burly of external life activity for a while.

6. Some people like to have an inspiring picture near them when they meditate -- of someone you love and respect, someone who symbolizes for you the state of inner peace and tranquility you want to contact.

7. Relax as much as you can beforehand, using the techniques suggested in this book. Then sit in a comfortable position, spine erect, chin parallel to the floor and tucked in slightly. Sitting cross-legged on the floor is best, or kneeling on a meditation bench. It is more important to be comfortable than to be correct, so if you need a chair, use one. If you use a chair, sit with both feet on the floor and arms by your sides, hands on thighs. Place your hands either palm-upwards on your thighs or lightly clasped in your lap. Make sure your shoulders are dropped back and relaxed, and your neck loose (rotate to relax). Begin, with closed eyes, to take long, slow, deep yogic breaths (see page 62).

Meditation on the Sound of "Om"

In this meditation, we practice focusing the mind on the sound of Om (rhymes with "home"). This sound is considered to be particularly relaxing and centering.

1. Close your eyes and sit quietly for a few minutes. Drop all expression from your face and consciously relax the various parts of your body, especially the face, shoulders, abdomen and hands.

2. Take long, deep breaths, using Yogic Deep Breathing (see p. 62). Continue this slow, deep breathing for 2-5 minutes and practice focusing your total concentration on the breaths. Then gradually allow your breath to return to normal and feel yourself becoming very still within. Try to feel rather than think.

3. Mentally repeat the sound of "Om" very slowly. Feel the vibrations of the thought. Listen with your whole being. Then, after several silent, mental repetitions of the sound, begin to very softly chant the sound aloud by taking a full, deep breath in and making the sound as you slowly exhale. Continue for a few minutes, making each repetition of the sound as long as is comfortably possible. Experience the effects. Feel the peace that is created by the vibration. Imagine that the sound is flowing from deep within the abdomen and you are opening up to let it flow out. Feel all worry, fear, and tension dissolve.

4. Remain still for a period of time, enjoying the feeling of quiet and peace within and around you. When you are ready, gradually open your eyes.

Practice this technique until you begin to feel that you are gaining some control and concentration, and then move onto a more complex technique.

"So-Hum", Internal Sound Meditation

So Hum, an easy but powerful technique, is also based on awareness of the breath and is one of the most scientific approaches for learning the deep concentration and inner stillness necessary to eventually experience meditation.

As with all techniques, take time to first arrange yourself in a comfortable easy-to-hold sitting position and consciously relax the various parts of your body. Allow your consciousness of external surroundings to fade as much as possible. Then practice a few minutes of Yogic Deep Breathing, focusing your attention on the breath.

1. After a few minutes (approximately 2-5) allow the breath to return to normal, gradually, but keep your concentration on it. Watch your normal flow of breath with unattached, objective awareness. Do not be tense or try to control your breathing in any way. Do not expect anything to happen. Just watch the breath flow in and out. You will notice that the breath will automatically begin to become slower and more shallow.

2. After a slow, gentle breathing rhythm is established, begin to picture, within, the sound of So-Hum ("I am that"). Do not actually make the sound, but imagine that it is the sound of the breath: Soooo on the inhalation and Hummmm on the exhalation. Let the breathing and the sound absorb your mind as completely as possible.

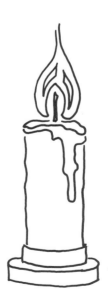

3. After a few weeks, add concentration on the point between the eyebrows (sometimes known as the "third eye"). Begin by practicing So Hum for about 10 minutes and gradually increase. Each time the mind wanders away from the technique, gently lead it back until the periods of mental stillness increase. A deep peacefulness will result.

Tratak - Visual Concentration

Tratak is commonly used as a meditation technique, although it is usually classified as a Yogic kriya (purification technique) because it also strengthens and improves the eyesight, and stimulates the brain cells and cranial nerves. It does, however, bring about the same benefits as other meditation techniques, in part because it develops concentration by exercising steadiness of gaze.

The following is a commonly used form of Tratak, Candle Gazing. It is especially useful for beginners.

1. Use a room that is quiet and dark, with little or no air currents.

2. Place a lighted candle at eye level, making sure that it is steady and can burn safely.

3. Sit straight in a chair or cross-legged on the floor so that the position is comfortable enough to hold with a minimum of movement. Consciously relax the body and mind, using a few minutes of deep breathing to help you relax (see previous techniques).

4. Begin to gaze steadily into the center of the flame. As your eyes begin to tire, close and relax them, visualizing the flame in the space between your eyebrows. You will actually see an image left by the flame. Concentrate on this image, without mental comment, until it fades completely. Then re-open your eyes and again gaze into the flame.

5. Repeat this alternate opening and closing of the eyes, concentrating completely on each phase and dropping all other thoughts from the mind. With practice, you will find that the mind will remain still for a longer period, even after the image has faded.

When your meditation time is over, keep the eyes closed for a few minutes and relax. A good technique for relaxing the eye muscles is to rub the palms together briskly until they feel hot, then lay them across your closed eyes until they cool again. The warmth from the palms will penetrate and relax the muscles of the eyes.

Begin by limiting your meditation time to 5 minutes, increasing it gradually as you become more adept at the technique.

HOW TO USE MEDITATION TO SOLVE PROBLEMS

Meditation is a profoundly effective way to solve all kinds of problems; indeed it is the most profound way for those who become familiar with how to use it. As we progress on the path of self-development we begin to understand more and more clearly, from our own experience, the yogic truth that the solution to *all* problems lies within us. At first this is not easy to believe, but practice of continual self-awareness and self-discovery techniques, such as the ones in this book, reveal, little by little, that the source of all our imagined problems lies within our own minds -- our own attitudes toward the world, our own habitual thinking patterns and motivations. In other words, we create our own experience of the world through *our* way of perceiving it.

Tapping the Unconscious for Solutions

This is a very exciting realization, because it also means that we ourselves have the power to resolve our problems and change our world. Yet these solutions are usually not at the level of the conscious mind. Like the paintings or poems of creative geniuses, creative solutions to life's problems tend to surface from deep within the unconscious without our conscious bidding. But even if we have no control over them, we are able to create circumstances which are favorable to their emergence. Deep physical and mental relaxation, and a calm mind relatively empty of thoughts, plans, and anxieties is the state in which solutions to problems will occur to us. This is

why meditation is such a powerful tool. The following method for internal problem-solving is based on the teachings of Yogi Desai.

When you have a difficulty with other people, it is better not to go to them immediately and talk about it. Wait until the immediate emotions have subsided. Projecting anger or negative emotions onto them is a great violence both to you and them. It is best to first use some form of inner processing *by yourself* to become clear about the things *in you* that have caused the problem. This introspection will enable you to do this objectively, without blaming either the other person, or yourself, simply seeing things as they are and taking responsibility (without guilt) for your part of the difficulty.

Step by Step Instructions

1. *First, write down your feelings* about the problem objectively and clearly to help you when you meditate. Ask yourself clear, specific questions. The more specific your questions, the more readily you'll come upon a solution. Look honestly at your feelings of pain, anger, fear, or whatever. Know that wherever there is pain, that is where your greatest attachment lies. Now ask yourself what your attachment is, what your desires are. You may use this same process during the meditation itself.

2. *Now, relax by* sitting comfortably and quietly in a relaxed position with your eyes closed. Relax yourself further by taking slow deep breaths for a few minutes.

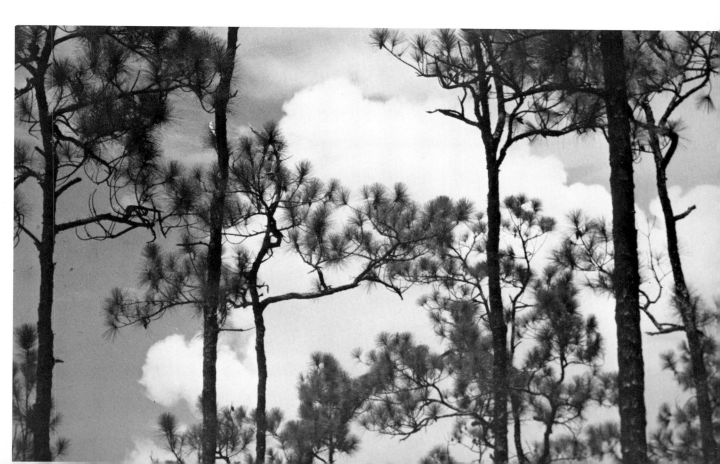

3. Begin to visualize, feel, or hear the voice of your own Inner Teacher or Guide. Everyone has such an Inner Teacher. He or she may be the image of an external person who provides you guidance or it may be someone you've never met (perhaps someone who is not even alive now) who nevertheless inspires you in moments of need or whose teachings you follow. It may simply be a voice, a feeling inside, a recognition of words of truth as they arise. Whatever it is, begin to feel an inner contact with this person or source of truth. Imagine yourself seated in conversation with him or her, if you wish (not everyone visualizes through images -- simply feeling it is another method).

4. Begin to ask your Inner Guide, "Teach me what the lesson is hidden in this situation. What can I learn?" Share your problem with your Inner Teacher, your Higher Self. Share it objectively and clearly. Feel the openness and acceptance of your Guide. At once you will feel clearer with your difficulty.

4. Hold in your conscious mind the thought-image of whatever you want to change. As you breathe in, watch the breath and the thought rising to the spot between the eyebrows (called the third eye) and dissolving. Do it over and over with each breath. This technique is especially effective during yogic breathing exercises.

5. Repeat this affirmation: "I am born divine; I have no problems. All of this is superficially imposed, artifically accepted because I have mistakenly believed in it. Now I am dropping and dissolving the problem. I no longer believe in it."

You may also wish to create another specific affirmation for yourself, to help you drop and dissolve a particular problem (see the next exercise for instructions).

6. Remain seated in meditation until you feel calmer and clearer about the situation on which you are processing. If one meditation does not enable you to feel completely clear and settled, then you may repeat the process as many times as you feel you need to become calm, clear and accepting of the situation. Affirmations, particularly, are very powerful when repeated consistently over a period of time.

Special Note

Sometimes when you process your feelings about a situation in this way, you may feel some strong emotions coming up. At this time, if you find it hard to channel that energy inwardly, you may want to find a place where you can safely express the feelings without directing them at someone else. Work out the feelings by beating a pillow or screaming into it, accepting that this is a natural

intermediate process until you can channel the feelings more internally. Caution: choose a place where you will not disturb others, or where they understand and accept what you are doing. A car with rolled up windows is pretty soundproof, or you can gain surprising relief from a 'silent scream' (going through the physical motions without making any actual sound). Another alternative, to change your energy and clear your head, is to take a cold shower and scream again (better let your family or roommates know what you're doing!)

Problem Solving During Kripalu Yoga Moving Meditation

As you learned earlier, Kripalu Yoga is a form of meditation while moving. As such, it can also be used for problem-solving in the following way:

When you are doing yoga postures in the Kripalu style, wherever you experience physical pain there is a corresponding psychological block related to it. Emotional and psychological resistances cause physical tension in related parts of the body (e.g. neck and shoulders) which in turn causes tensed muscles that create a barrier to the flow of energy. This is where the pain is felt, as those cramped muscles are stretched and the energy tries to push its way through. So concentrate on relaxing the muscles in that painful area. Try to relate the physical area that is painful to an emotional or psychological difficulty that you know you have. As you hold the posture, consciously send relaxation to that area and visualize your psychological block dissolving as the muscles relax.

HOW TO PRACTICE CREATIVE VISUALIZATION & AFFIRMATION

We do not realize how suggestible and easy to influence our subconscious mind is. As a result we seldom use that suggestibility in a positive, creative way to change our own lives. Instead, we are constantly influencing the way we feel by our negative reinforcements and thoughts ("I can't...I've never been able to...I'm not the kind of person who...I wish I could...If only I...", etc.) Our subconscious mind is like a child which listens to these thoughts and is influenced and formed by them. Simple everyday examples can show us how this is true. For example, you're carrying a pile of dishes and you start to think: "Oh dear, what if I should drop one?" -- and next thing, you do! Or you're skiing and you see a rock or tree in the way, and you think: "I hope I don't hit that tree." No sooner have you thought that than you seem to head straight towards that very tree! We can all come up with numerous examples.

Harnessing our Thought Energy

This "influence-ability" of the subconscious can be a tremendous blessing, as well as a curse, if we know how to use it. The Kripalu Approach uses a technique called "Creative Visualization and Affirmation", which harnesses the power of thought energy for growth and change. By visualizing, in your mind's eye, the situation as you would like to see it unfold, or yourself as you would like to be, you are creating a new formative influence on yourself to replace the old one. This influence will be as powerful as the energy of belief you put into it. If you believe it won't work,

it won't, because you won't be putting enough energy into the visualization/affirmation for it to impress itself on your subconscious. Thoughts are energy (it is important to understand this) and energy has power.

It is important to understand, too, that you are not "whistling in the dark" or going through a "pie-in-the-sky" routine by trying to make yourself believe something that is, in actual fact, not true. Affirmation is different from hypnotic suggestion. What you are affirming *is* already true. Your true Inner Self (as distinct from your physical, material self) is a perfect blueprint. You already *are* fearless, balanced, loving, contented, right now on the deepest levels of your being. Layers of blocks have simply come between the self and you, so that the blueprint has not been perfectly executed in material form in the body and mind. In your affirmation (for example: "I am fearless") you are speaking the absolute truth. You are the voice of the spiritual Self speaking to your material self, your body-mind. When you can accept and believe this, you can start to make affirmations and visualizations really work for you and affect great changes in your life.

Moshe Feldenkrais, originator of the Feldenkrais Technique for body integration, has demonstrated that when people rehearse a physical action in their minds they perform it as well as, or even better than, when they have physically practiced the same action.

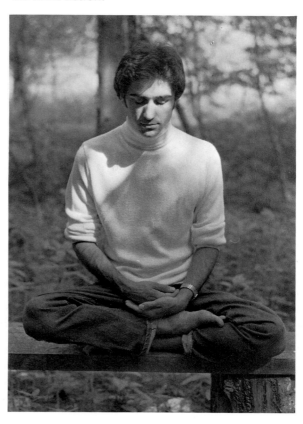

The Technique

1. Select one area in which you would like to make changes such as:
  (a) to be more relaxed
  (b) to have calmer emotions when dealing with difficulties
  (c) to be more accepting of yourself
  (d) to worry less
  (e) to lead a healthier life

2. Deeply relax your body and mind, using the techniques outlined earlier in this book.

3. Begin to see yourself in your mind's eye, as if someone were looking at you. Picture yourself as you will be when you have changed in the way you want. See it very vividly and in detail. See yourself going through a specific situation with the actions you will perform and the thoughts and feelings you will have, when you are that changed person. See and feel other people responding to that changed you. Feel it with great intensity. Enjoy the experience deeply, as if it were really happening.

4. Choose an affirmation that expresses this area in which you would like to change, and repeat it several times, aloud if possible (if not, then mentally). Make the affirmation very simple, short and specific. For example: "I am a capable and loveable person and I like myself" or "It is OK to make mistakes; I accept myself when I make a mistake."

5. Work on one simple and specific area until you feel you have made progress before trying another one.

6. Always be very positive when you practice affirmation, selecting your words carefully. Avoid thinking of visualizing the problems, the difficulties, the "down" side. You will only reinforce them. Stay with the positive side.

7. Avoid the trap of feeling justified in your experience of the problem situation you are trying to change. The point is not to change the situation or the other people. Even if you could, you'd still have to face the same problem over again the next time the problem came up. Even though you may be "right", if your attitude to the situation/conflict disturbs your inner peace why hold onto the attitude? If you are driving up to an intersection and have a green traffic light, but someone who has a red light is obviously not going to stop, you'd be crazy to go ahead even though you have the right of way! So seek to do what will give *you* peace of mind, no matter what happens. Find where changing your own attitude can change the way you experience the world.

8. Believe that the technique of affirmation can work for you. This is very important. It is perhaps hard for the rational mind to accept this, as it is a new concept for many people. Yet more and more, science and psychology are coming to make discoveries about the workings of the unconscious mind which support this technique. Most of us have come to accept the fact that our unconscious minds can be "programed" to respond in certain ways with certain behavior. Hypnotism rests on this fact. What we perhaps have not yet realized is that who and what we are is a result of all the programing that *we,* ourselves, have accomplished by our unconscious thinking patterns all our lives.

Reversing Our Programing

We have to undo this programing where it has had negative results. We must consciously affirm a positive thought to replace each negative one, and also repeat that positive thought enough times that it erases the deeply-imprinted negative thought which we have been unconsciously "affirming" throughout our lives.

For this reason, it is often helpful to not only think a positive affirmation, but also to write it down, a number of times, since this involves several of the senses at once. It is also helpful to observe the negative responses or resistances that come up in your mind as you write the affirmations and to write them down too. See the appendix for further books to read on affirmations.

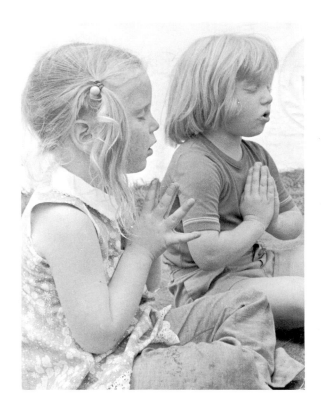

SPIRITUAL ATTUNEMENT IN DAILY LIFE

Meditation, as we have just seen, is an essential part of a holistically healthy lifestyle, because it helps us to be more attuned to our prana, to our inner spiritual self. The next step is extending the all-too-brief experience of meditation into our daily lives so that we become more attuned to prana ongoingly. In this way we will become more relaxed, balanced, flowing and centered in whatever we do.

In actual fact, we are already doing this to some extent in our lives. Whenever we are totally immersed in something we love doing -- dancing, singing, painting, gardening -- we are experiencing a form of meditation or spiritual attunement because our body, mind and prana are all united and harmonized in the activity. These experiences, however, are few and far between for most of us. Normally we are doing one thing with our bodies while our minds are off in a totally different direction and our prana is forgotten entirely. We are not conscious of *who* we are, of the reality and supremacy of our inner Self. We go through the day mechanically, for the most part. In the singing-dancing-gardening experience just mentioned, we are also not consciously attuning to prana, yet spontaneously we are experiencing a harmony of all parts of our being. The ideal is to bring about this harmony consciously and constantly. The following article by Yogi Desai explains how to do this by practicing different kinds of awareness throughout the day.

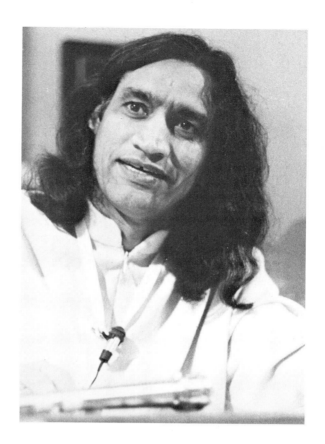

THE MEDITATION OF PRANA LIVING

by Yogi Amrit Desai

The purpose of applying the techniques of Kripalu Yoga to everyday life is to become more and more sensitive and attuned to your prana. Then every movement and thought becomes harmonious and relaxed, and your whole life becomes a meditation. This is the meditation of prana living.

How can you do this? By applying each individual stage of Kripalu Yoga to your daily life and bringing the same awareness and concentration to your everyday movements as you do to a yoga posture. We perform yoga postures with awareness and attention because they are different from how we move in everyday life; they are special, unusual. Most people perform their normal, daily activities, however, in a mechanical way. They have no awareness of what they are doing or how they are doing it, because the actions required are familiar, habitual. Kripalu Yoga will help you break this mechanicalness and become fully conscious and aware of each action. Then you can choose to perform only those actions which are necessary, in a way that is harmonious with your prana. By doing this, you will multiply the energy you have at your disposal and remain deeply relaxed no matter what you are doing. This is "the meditation of prana living" -- the highest, most holistic way of life.

Stage 1 -- Body Postures

First, Become Aware of Your Posture and Relax

The first stage of Kripalu Yoga is perfecting the postures, but formal postures are only one medium of expression for Kripalu Yoga. If you raise your hands in a certain way it can be an expression of Kripalu Yoga also. The first way to use your knowledge of Kripalu Yoga is to become aware of the many different "postures" you assume throughout the day.

Right now, just freeze where you are. You are in a "posture". You will change that posture often throughout the day to fit the needs of your body. This will be automatically regulated by your prana (if you don't block it by lack of attunement) rather than by your conscious mind. As much as possible during the day, become aware of how prana, as expressed in the feelings in your body, wants to regulate your posture. Then follow its guidance. Move, sit and stand in the way that feels good to your body, whenever practical. Of course there are places where you cannot assume the posture that feels best to you. For example, your prana may tell you to lie down, but if you are in your office you probably can't do that! At such times, simply maintain whatever posture is appropriate, but do it with relaxed awareness. Then, even if you cannot follow your prana you are at least more aware of its needs.

If you always remain aware of your posture, you will be very relaxed and prana will always flow freely through your body. Awareness of your body position and relaxation through the day, as often as you can remember, is practicing Kripalu Yoga, Step One, all day long. Whenever you become fully conscious of your body position, you will immediately experience relaxation and a flow of energy because you are listening to your prana much more closely than before. You will become extremely aware of your own presence, your form, your communication with your body and your surroundings. This is how Kripalu Yoga postures can help to increase your awareness all day long. Do whatever you are doing with awareness, in a very relaxed way, and notice how much tension you drop when you consciously relax your movements. In other words, be conscious as often as you can while you are doing different things during the day. For example, be aware of how the natural flow of energy is carrying you when you walk, and you will see the difference. Or, if you are changing your clothes, become aware of every position you assume. You'll be amazed at what happens to you. You'll be changing postures, and these postures will be unique when you do them with consciousness. Normally you move your body in many different positions all day long, but hardly ever with con-scious awareness. Kripalu Yoga is a method of interjecting awareness into every mechanical action that you are performing. That is very powerful.

Second, Change Your Posture to Change Your Mood

The second way to use postures in everyday life is to learn to assume the proper posture once you are aware that your posture is incorrect. Each posture expresses a certain feeling, and correcting it will change how you feel. For example, if you are feeling depressed or frustrated, become aware of how you are walking. You walk in a different way. Your back begins to slump, your head droops a little so that you are looking down at the ground rather than straight ahead. At such times, use your awareness to pull up your physical center of gravity which is pulling you down emotionally. Consciously straighten and walk tall. Now, again, you are using Kripalu Yoga, because Kripalu Yoga is one way of not letting your emotions take over your mind. Instead, constantly attune your mind to your prana, to your Higher Self, and use posture to lift yourself out of negative feelings through conscious awareness. When you are feeling depressed, anxious, frustrated or any other negative emotion, just correct your posture and walk straight, in a relaxed way, and see what happens.

Dress, too, has an important influence on how you feel. Never allow yourself to dress in an ugly or shabby way, especially when you're not feeling good. Instead, take a bath or shower, put on clean clothes and then walk out with your head held high. Even put on an artificial smile if you have to. You are not being dishonest, because you are doing it consciously for a specific, good purpose. In other words, if you haven't enough control yet over your inner mechanisms to simply feel good, take the support of every external means in your power. As you create a positive vibration all around you, other people will begin to feed you positive energy in return, and this will also help to change your energy. There is nothing "phoney" about this, because you are doing it consciously. You are not doing it mechanically or for any false motivation. You are not trying to hide anything. You are simply consciously using every means at your disposal to come out of a negative experience.

Third: Let Your Thoughts Follow Your Posture

There is a third way you can use the postures and positions of your body to heighten your con-sciousness. Some examples will best describe it. When you are reclining, consciously recline and feel deeply rested. Don't think about something else which involves sitting up and walking. When you are sitting, just sit there. Have you seen a cat when it is resting? It just lies there, totally relaxed, and yet, when it wants to jump, it moves like lightning. So be like a cat: when you are sitting, sit with your mind too. When you are walking, walk. When you are lying, lie down. When you are working, work. In other words, your posture will help you to get in touch with wherever you are and to stay grounded in it, to fully accept it. It will help you to bring your mind and body into harmony.

Have you noticed people who, when they are sitting and talking to you, always look as if they are ready to leap to their feet? They spend almost as much energy as if they were actually running, and this is a waste. Often when people are sitting, they are thinking of doing something else, and so there is a split between the mind and the body. The thoughts in the mind are at variance with the posture, causing the body to lose a lot of energy. If you use your posture for awareness, by bringing your thoughts into harmony with your body position, you will be able to cut off all that unnecessary wastage of energy. As a result, you will be relaxed and your energy will always be very high. You'll be able to do whatever you want to do very effectively.

In Summary: Use Posture To Attune To Prana

In other words, use yoga postures as an example of how to consciously attune your thoughts to your body. This will enable you to be more relaxed, yet alert. In this way, you are living more naturally, according to the higher energy of prana rather than the false, restless energy of the individual mind and ego.

Many people are impressed by the marvelous achievements of those who are prominent in their fields. Yet often, I am not impressed. I see that most of the time they draw their energy from ego. All their accomplishments are for the rest of the world and maybe for history, but not for themselves. What good is it when you have all the external accomplishments and everybody else says how wonderful you are, but you don't feel wonderful? Inside you feel unsatisfied, unfulfilled, or unhealthy. Kripalu Yoga teaches you how to become more fulfilled by attuning to prana, and becoming free of the grip of the ego. Awareness of body postures is an important beginning.

Stage 2 -- Using the Breath

The second way to use Kripalu Yoga to attune to prana is to become aware of your breathing during the day. Right now, become aware of how you are breathing. Feel your breath flowing in and out. You are again making contact with your prana, this time through your breath. You are again becoming fully aware of your body in

relation to the surrounding elements. Life is coming to you as physical experience rather than as thoughts. Your body is the only medium that you have to experience life. This awareness will also make your mind very centered, so that it can really take in the experience. As soon as you attend to your breath and regulate it, extraneous thoughts will instantly leave, and you will be able to concentrate on what you are experiencing in that moment.

Whenever you are emotional, your breathing becomes shallow and irregular. As soon as you become aware of it, you will automatically want to breathe more deeply, regularly and slowly, because this is the natural way of breathing. This is how children and animals at rest breathe. When you breathe slowly and deeply, you are taking in more prana from the air, and you are balancing your mind and emotions. Almost instantly, you will feel a calmness creeping over you. After you have practiced this for a while, you will begin to experience a real sense of mastery over your emotions. You will know that no outside force needs to affect you -- that your reactions are all within your own control. It will change your entire life.

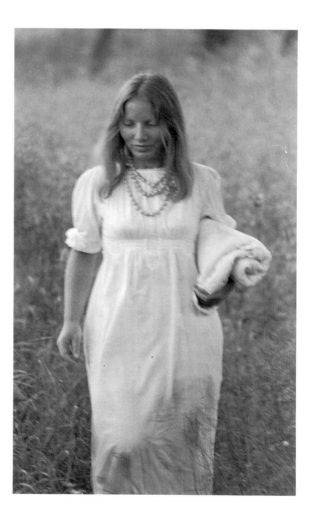

You will eventually become able to control every little thought that goes through you, every little emotion. You will know exactly what to do and what not to do at any given time. You will know what things you don't want to do, and you will be able to stop doing them. For example, suppose you don't want to overeat. Conscious awareness of your body through posture and breathing will enable you to stop eating at just the right time. The awareness will give you that control.

You will also accumulate tremendous amounts of energy by breath awareness. Not only do you breathe in more energy, you also dissipate less energy by getting less emotional. So breath awareness, as taught in Kripalu Yoga, is another way of establishing yourself in prana consciousness.

Stage 3 -- Slow Down and Be With Your Speed

In the third stage of Kripalu Yoga, the body postures are done in extremely slow motion. To practice this in your daily life, simply slow down everything that you do. Give yourself time for everything. If you are putting on your shirt, do it in slow motion. When you are putting on your shoes, do it very slowly and consciously. Allow your actions to come from your conscious awareness, rather than from mechanical habits. This awareness will help you to change your habits. Even if you just seem to be going from one habit to another, that's fine. The next one is at least a new habit and, in the meanwhile, you have learned a new awareness: how to change your old habits. Human beings are creatures of habit. Until we are enlightened, we still will have some habits. But more awareness is necessary, and this technique of slowing down in everything is helpful. For example, every time you get into your car, there is a specific, habitual way you do it. Consciously change the way you get in. For example, sit down first, and then swing in both of your legs very gracefully. This is the whole point of slowing down: to perform every movement gracefully and flowingly with no hitch, no jerk, no suddenness. This conserves energy. The slowness of the movement brings another kind of awareness to everything that you do. Slow down, or even stop before you start something. If you are driving a car, for example, and you are in the habit of always driving at seventy miles an hour, stop and consciously ask yourself if you *really* want and need to drive that fast. First, become aware of the tension created by the attention you have to pay and by the fear of being caught. Time your journey and see how much time you actually save by going at seventy miles an hour, as opposed to fifty-five miles an hour. If you save seven minutes, ask yourself this question: "Is all this tension worth it, to save seven minutes?" Then consciously intervene and slow down your driving.

The second technique is to think slow when you are *being* slow. Be with your speed. When you are driving at fifty-five miles an hour, which is the normal speed limit, consciously accept your speed of fifty-five and don't wish you were going at seventy -- because then you will experience a fifteen-mile-an-hour tension. Use your slowness to become conscious of your habits and to change them. Whether you are talking or walking, consciously slow down. Slow down your speech, and listen to it. Slow down your walking and feel every movement. As soon as you slow down, your prana will take over. You will move from consciousness, rather than from the mechanical part of your mind. You'll feel very relaxed, because when you slow down, you automatically drop into a relaxed state, into your feeling center, your prana. It happens spontaneously, when you slow down, you don't have to know how to do it. Your consciousness comes alive at once. Your awareness comes alive. Slowing down is a powerful way to train your consciousness.

Stage 4 -- Affirming Life

The fourth stage of Kripalu Yoga is holding the posture, accompanied by creative visualization. To use this in everyday life observe clearly everything you are doing and make it into an affirmation. For example, right now, as you read, consciously affirm and acknowledge to yourself: "I am enjoying these teachings thoroughly; they are speaking directly to my heart, and they are transforming my life. They are going very deep into me."

Using affirmations ongoingly in your life means being consciously aware, at every moment, of the good things that are happening to you and acknowledging them. So often we let the good things slip by us, taking them for granted, yet when unpleasant things are happening we become very conscious of them and complain loudly. Affirm the good things that are already happening to you. (This is what makes Kripalu affirmations very different from suggestion or self-hypnosis, in which you try to convince yourself of something which is not actually happening.) This technique can be applied all day long, like the others. For example, if you are in a traffic jam and you can't go any faster, just sit back, relax your posture, and acknowledge: "There is nothing I can do at this time, so here I am and that's fine. I'll take advantage of the situation to relax." That's your affirmation -- simply acknowledging and accepting exactly what is happening, without frustration.

Prana affirmations are those made within the

scope of existing conditions and situations. In following prana you are not trying to change the existing situation, you are learning to flow with it. You are simply affirming it, by being consciously aware of the good side of what is happening, and verbally acknowledging it, either mentally or aloud. It is such a simple technique, yet it can change your life. You will have so much energy by the end of the day. Usually you are tired because you spend so much energy by mentally fighting things that cannot be changed, by not accepting what is.

Stage 5 - Flowing with Life

The Heart of the Kripalu Approach

Finally, the fifth stage of Kripalu Yoga is the posture flow. If you practice all the awarenesses outlined here, throughout the day, you will begin to experience yourself flowing through life. Whether things happen the way you want or whether they don't, you will just flow through it, accepting everything. You will not resist anything, mentally or emotionally. You will not fight anything. You will always work with it, not against it. Your mind will become very clear. You will just have to ask yourself: "What is the next thing that I need to do?" Then you will be able to do it effortlessly. You will never be clogged by thoughts from previous moments. You will be fresh every moment because your mind is in harmony with your prana. You will do what you need to do, not what will fulfill the dreams of the ego. You will sleep when you are sleepy and eat when you are hungry; you will rest when you are tired. You will follow whatever messages come naturally from prana. You will flow with life, always content, always relaxed. This is the Kripalu Approach to life. This is the meditation of prana living.

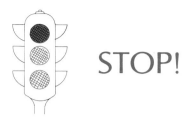

STOP!

STOP! How aware are you of your body's messages *right now*? How are you feeling? Is there tension, stiffness, tiredness in any part of your body? Do you need to get up and stretch? Take some deep breaths? Relax your shoulders? Rest your eyes? Rest your mind? Close your eyes for a minute and take some long, slow deep breaths to enable you to get in touch with your experience. Then respond to what your body is asking you to do.

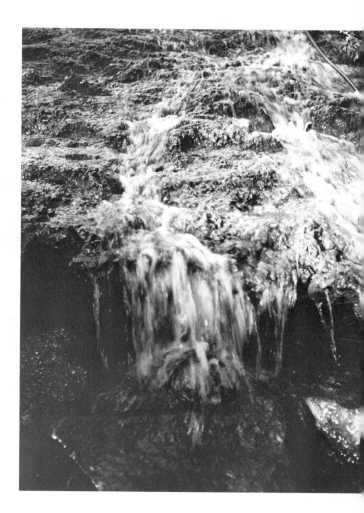

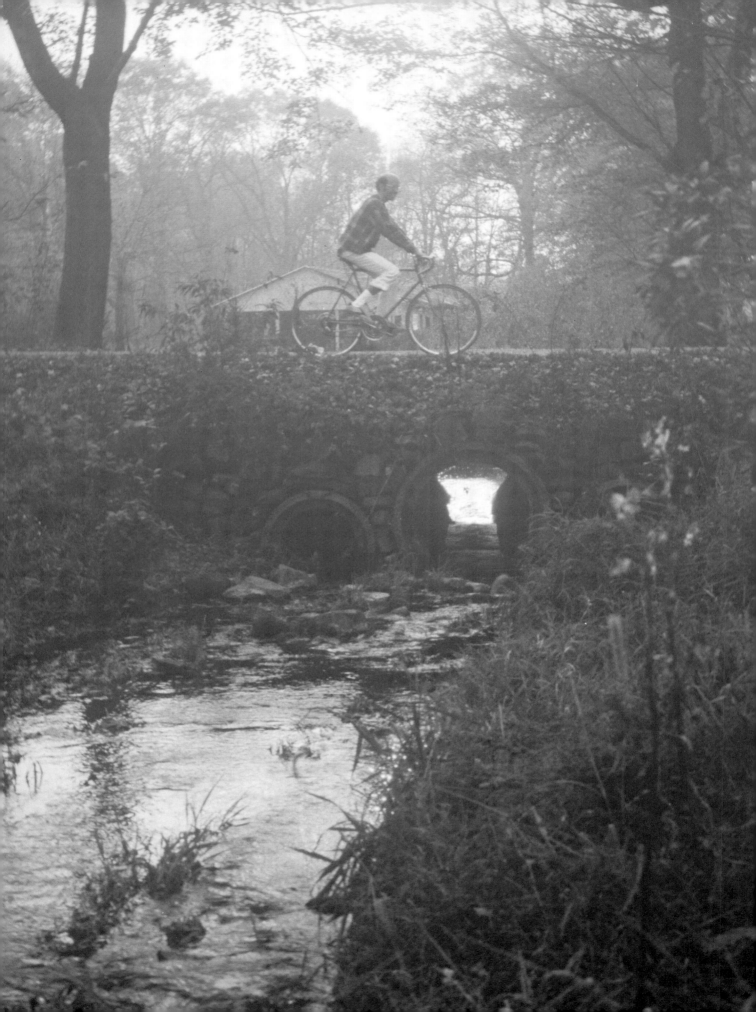

WAY EIGHT
creating a supportive lifestyle

HOLISTIC HEALTH INVOLVES YOUR WHOLE LIFE

It will have become clear to you by now that the Kripalu Approach is more than simply a group of new techniques that can be added to your lifestyle. It is, in fact, a lifestyle in itself, a whole new way of living. It proposes that, in the words of Yogi Amrit Desai: "You can't change your life without involving your life in the change." In other words, we have come full circle, back to where we started at the beginning of the book: *Holistic* Health is the sum of how you live your *whole* life. This chapter explores the following questions: "How well does my present lifestyle support my aspiration for health and wholeness of body, mind and spirit?" and "How can I modify my lifestyle so that it becomes more supportive of these aspirations?"

There are three major elements involved in creating a supportive lifestyle, so this chapter is broken into three sections to cover each one separately. They are:

A. Your own actions

B. Your environment

C. Your relationships

In reality, of course, these elements are not separate but interdependent. For instance, the people you relate to are both a consequence of and a part of your environment. Yet each area is a distinct element of support, without which any lifestyle change would be incomplete. You may seem to be doing all the right things for your life that are within your power, but if your environment is inconsistent with your needs and aspirations, your progress will be limited. Conversely, you may be in a totally supportive environment,

but if your actions are not geared towards nurturing your own health, you will not benefit much. And if your relationships with others are not harmonious and appropriate, again your growth will be held back.

"The Eighth Way", then, is geared towards helping you understand (a) how your activities, your relationships and your environment influence your health and well-being and (b) how these may need to be modified in specific ways to bring your lifestyle more into harmony with your health goals. This is not, however, a chapter on self-denial and deprivation! We are talking about changes that you yourself decide you *want* to make, not things you feel you "should" do but don't want to. The path to Holistic Health is always a joyful one because we are making our own choices. To again quote Yogi Desai: "A life of Holistic Health is not a giving-up life; it is simply knowing what you really want." So here, to begin with, is the area over which you have the greatest immediate control: your own personal actions and activities.

YOUR ACTIVITIES

To begin this section, first review each of the Self-Discovery Experiences you have completed, with particular attention to the first one, "Check Your Holistic Health Quotient." See what you have learned from each one, in terms of how well your actions and activities contribute to your experience of health and harmonious body-mind-spirit integration. Notice how you *feel* about each area of activity -- how interested you are in working on that area, how much it appeals to you, how much you would enjoy it and find it fun, or whether you feel you are not ready for it yet. Pay particular attention to the "Adjustment" sections, where you have outlined possible ways to change what you are doing.

Now you are ready for action! Probably you have ongoingly been implementing some of these techniques into your daily life. The next step is to develop an integrated, balanced plan of action, so that you do not take on too much and become discouraged, or concentrate too much in one area and create new imbalances to replace the old ones. The first and most important step is to set priorities: to establish what is most important to you and the order in which you want to proceed. The following chart will help you.

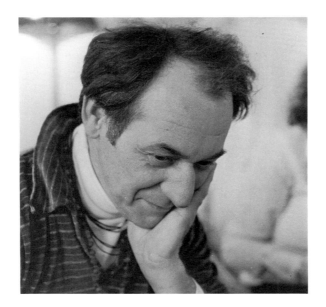

Setting Priorities

Go down the following list of possible growth objectives and place an "A" in the appropriate box which indicates the priority of that objective for you. Try not to evaluate these objectives in terms of what you think you *should* do but in terms of what you *want* to do and what would *feel* good to you to work on.

	Top Priority	Very Important	Important, but can wait	Not right now
1. Improving my diet				
2. Getting more exercise				
3. Taking up yoga				
4. Adjusting my sleep/rest habits for greater regularity				
5. Taking relaxation daily				
6. Establishing group support for health practices and spiritual activity				
7. Regular self-observation through journal, introspection or other means				
8. Regular use of cleansing diet, fasting and purification				
9. Beginning to meditate				
10. Cultivating more relaxed, harmonious relationships and attitudes at work				
11. Allowing the child in me more room for creativity and play				
12. Improving my communications and relationships with my friends and family				
13. Achieving greater inner attunement				
14. Other (you list)				

_____

_____

Developing A Growth Plan: How Do I Go About Making the Changes I Desire?

A. Now that you have set your priorities for growth, go back over your list of top priority growth items and pick *one* that you especially want to focus on in the immediate future. If you did not have any top priority items then choose from the "very important" items.

In choosing your growth goal, don't pick something that you *know* would be very difficult to change. For example, you may want to eat moderately but also know that it is too much to expect of yourself right now, given everything else that is going on in your life.

Choose something that you feel you could change with a moderate amount of effort and concentration. For example, you may decide that taking relaxation on a daily basis is a growth goal that is within your capacity to accomplish right now. Once having mastered relaxation, you will be in a better position to make a direct change in your eating habits.

B. After choosing your priority, make a very specific list of all of the possible ways you could go about acquiring this new habit. In the case of taking daily relaxation, you might list:
I could practice: before lunch for 15 minutes
before dinner for 15 minutes
in the bus to and from work
as I wait for meetings to begin
as I stand in line at the lunch counter, etc.

C. Go over this list and pick the one approach to change that is most *practical* and *realistic* for you to have some degree of success with, given your current life conditions. You may decide to practice relaxation everyday before lunch, because you know that relaxing before dinner is impossible with the kids and the dog around.

D. Choose a length of time (one or two weeks) to practice this new behavior, with the goal of reviewing how you are doing at the end of that time. It helps to keep a daily journal of your experiences in acquiring your new skill. A sample entry might read "tried relaxation for 12 minutes today in office but was interrupted by secretary -- will have to put 'do not disturb' note on my door tomorrow". As you make entries, you learn how you are doing and your journal becomes a record of your accomplishments and joys in growth.

E. Most important of all, as you embark on your journey learn to cultivate an attitude of acceptance of yourself and whatever happens. Whenever we try something new, we meet our own inner resistance. There is a part of every one of us that wants to grow and change, and be a better person, And there is also a hidden part of us that, deep down, doesn't want to, that prefers the ease and security of our present known habits and way of life, that fears the unknown, or is simply lazy! We can only overcome this resistance by first accepting it (ourselves) and learning to work with and through it. Everything that happens to us can enhance our awareness and, consequently, our joy of living if we *accept* it. Remember the THREE A's FORMULA TO WELL-BEING: If I'm AWARE of who I am, and I ACCEPT the self I see, then I'll have all I'll ever need to ADJUST to become the REAL ME.

Remain inspired: In order to change your unhelpful health habits, you will need to constantly re-inspire yourself to be consistent in your efforts. Consult the book and tape resources listed in the appendix so that you may continue to be full of enthusiasm for the journey you are undertaking.

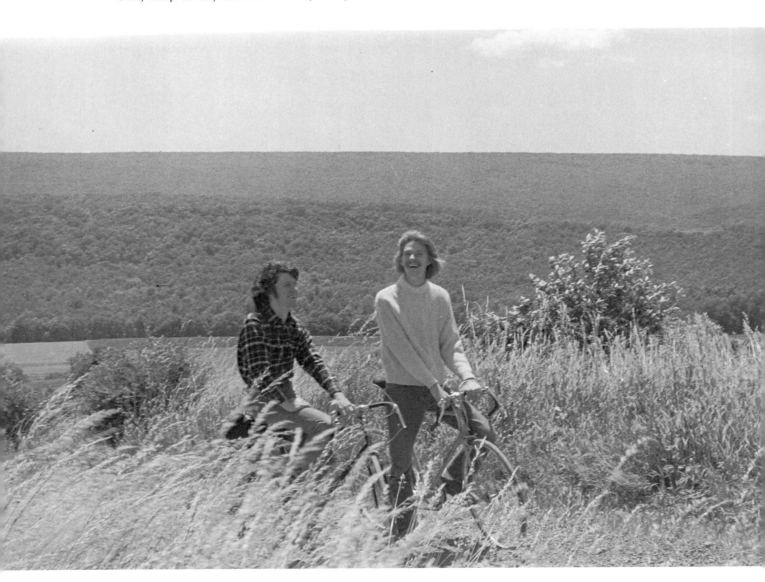

YOUR ENVIRONMENT

The Surroundings

Now that you have decided on a specific plan of action for your daily activities, let's take a look at your environment, or more accurately, your environments, for you pass through many different environments even in one day.

The dictionary defines "environment" as follows: "The external conditions in which a *person or organism* lives." Well, it's obvious that you are a person living in an environment, but have you thought of yourself as an "organism"? This implies something that is vital, sensitive and easily affected by external conditions. An organism takes in and is nourished by the things that surround it. Remember learning in biology about the life of a simple cell and how it takes in nutrients through a process of absorption called osmosis? Now reflect on the fact that your body is nothing more or less than a vast conglomeration of millions of cells, which are constantly absorbing "nutrients" from their environment, and you will begin to understand better just how sensitive your body is.

How does this absorption happen? Principally through the medium of the five senses; not only are we hearing, seeing, tasting and smelling the world around us, we are also feeling it with every inch of our skin.

YOUR SURROUNDINGS ARE SPIRITUAL "FOOD"

Another important characteristic of a living organism is that it constantly adapts to its environment. This is how the whole process of evolution happens. In the same way, the human body is constantly being called upon to adjust and adapt

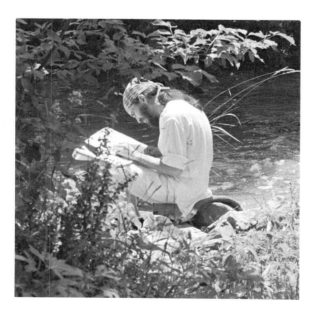

to its surroundings. It is important for our health that these physiological adaptations be in the right direction; that is, that the adaptation required be one favorable to health. The same is true for the impressions created by external stimuli; just as we need to be careful of what food we eat to nourish our bodies, so too we need to be aware and careful of what impressions we allow ourselves to take in. Since our senses tend not to discriminate, but to take in all that surrounds them, whether or not we are aware of it, it follows that we must be very discriminating in terms of the environments in which we allow ourselves to be.

This is where we have to decide what is supportive, in terms of environment, and what is not. To return again to the dictionary, supportive means: "that which holds or props up; provides for the needs of; helps, approves of; encourages." So, a supportive environment is one which provides for the needs of the organism -- your body, mind and spirit -- and encourages your total growth.

Picture yourself for a moment standing on a busy downtown street. Cars are rushing by, horns are honking, exhaust fumes fill the air, people walk briskly past, litter lines the sidewalk, buildings tower above you, a myriad of neon signs invite you to buy this and try that, the smell of hot pretzels from a nearby vendor drifts past your nose, someone on the square opposite is making a speech to the crowd about nuclear energy…all of these impressions bombarding your senses are asking for an adjustment from the body; an adaptation, a movement, an action, or a reaction. This means that they are all placing an energy demand on the body. No wonder, then, that the city dweller is often tired when he gets home.

NOURISH YOURSELF WITH HEALTHFUL SURROUNDINGS

Now visualize yourself in the country, walking along a tree-lined lane amidst quiet fields. All you hear are birds twittering, the occasional bark of a dog, and perhaps a distant chain-saw as the only sound of civilization. You are breathing fresh, cool air and the gentle breeze caresses your skin…

These examples are not given to condemn city life and tell everyone to move to the country, but rather to illustrate a subtle point and to aid your awareness so that you can balance out the environments you are in. The more external stimuli, the greater the energy demand on the body. The more unhealthy the surroundings, the more the body is called on to adapt. In the first visualization, chances are you felt yourself tensing slightly to combat the noise and fumes. In the second, you probably felt yourself relaxing. Relaxation is a free-flowing energy, as we have seen, and tension is blockage and waste of energy.

Our environment is absolutely key to the Kripalu Approach, which teaches that conserving our prana energy and being relaxed will lead us to Holistic Health. A truly supportive environment feeds our senses with its harmony, order and peace. It could be a quiet country setting, but it could also be a homey kitchen redolent with the smell of lovingly-prepared food. It could be a circle of old friends sharing their happiness and sorrow; a tidy desk with an inspiring picture; a simply furnished meditation room in harmonious, quiet colors; a brisk walk to work through pre-trafficed streets...these are just a few simple examples of a supportive environment, one in which you can feel peaceful, at ease, relaxed and in tune with the needs of your inner being.

The Social Aspect of Environment

It is not only our physical environment which affects us, it is also the people with whom we interact in that environment or environments. This means that we must also consider the people we spend time with (and how we spend that time) in terms of how they contribute to our growth. This is not a way to advocate selfishness -- at least, not in the usual sense of the word (see the following section on Relationships). It is rather an invitation to seriously evaluate whether certain social situations are really supportive of your health ideals and, if not, what to do about them.

Perhaps some examples will make this a little clearer. Let's say you have decided you want to eat a more natural, wholesome, healthy diet, free of refined, processed foods containing chemical additives. If you usually find yourself eating meals with a group of people with different needs and awarenesses, who prefer what you regard as unhealthy, nutritionless food, you will experience conflicting desires and a resultant energy loss. You want to be with them, or at least not to lose their friendship, yet you feel badly when you eat what you know is not good for you. The same thing will happen if you prefer not to drink alcohol, yet you spend a lot of time with people who like to go to bars; or if you've given up smoking and yet many situations involve your being in smoke-filled environments. Of course, you may not always seem to have a choice. If you work in an office where everyone smokes, it might seem to be a no-choice situation. On the other hand, you can always stop and ask yourself: "Do I have a choice? Could I work somewhere else? What is most important to me?"

With this idea of choice in mind, complete the Self-Discovery Experience which follows to see if it will reveal to you some new choices you can make to create a more supportive environment.

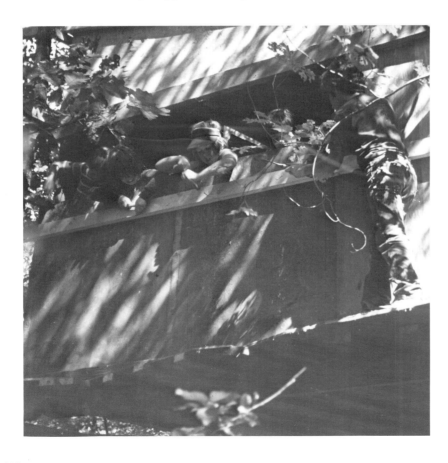

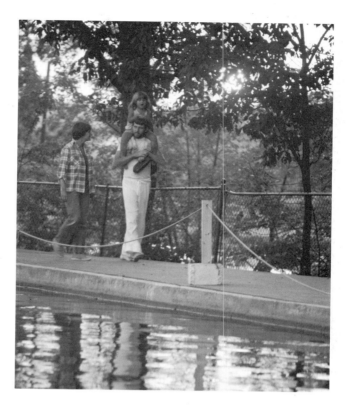

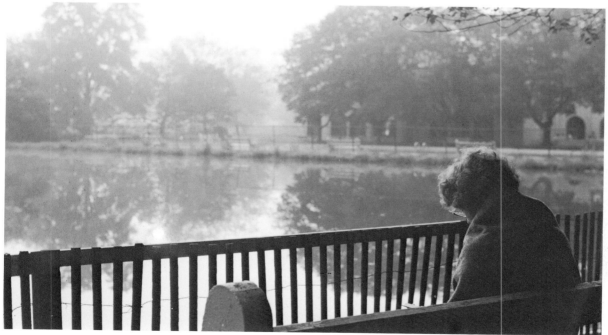

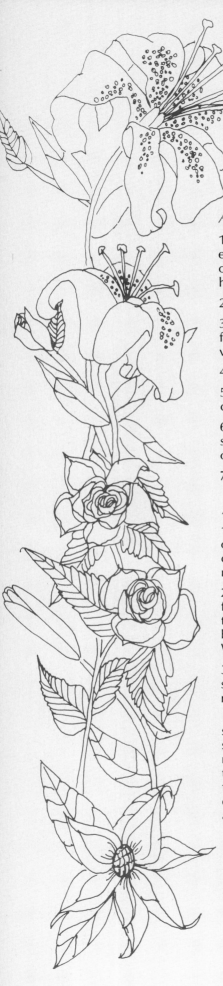

Self-Discovery

How Well Does Your Environment Support Your Health?

Awareness

1. Sit quietly and reflect for a moment with your eyes closed. Review all the different environments in which you find yourself in the course of a typical day. List *everything* on a sheet of paper, starting with your bed when you wake and passing through your house, your car, the subway, etc., until the last thing at night.

2. Circle the environments you like best and which support your growth.

3. Look over the circled items. Close your eyes and visualize yourself in each one for a few minutes. Really experience it. See and feel the people and the setting, hear the voices, taste the tastes, smell the odors.

4. After each visualization, list the *feelings* that came up in you.

5. Now reflect on and write down what it is that your favorite environments have in common. In what ways are they similar?

6. Think for a moment about the people in those environments. List the people. Describe how you feel about them, the quality of the time you spend with them, the level of communication between you.

7. Circle the people you enjoy being with, who also support your health and growth.

Acceptance

1. Take a look at the environments and people you didn't circle. Ask yourself for each one: "Do I wish to avoid these environments, people, situations? If so, do I have a choice -- can I avoid it/them? Why don't I, if I can? What do I stand to lose? What do I need from these environments, situations, and people? How else can I meet that need?"

2. Select one of these environments where you experience conflicting needs and feelings. Enter into it, with your eyes closed, through creative visualization. Explore those needs and feelings. Ask yourself: "What do I really want in my life? How can I best achieve it through this situation? What is pulling me away from my main purpose? Why do I allow it?"

3. Now for the other situations which seem not to be good for your Holistic Health and spiritual growth, ask yourself: "What other needs am I trying to meet? Are these needs really important to me? If they are, how else can I meet them?"

You will probably see that in many such situations the underlying need is either social (to have fun, companionship, friendship) or relaxation. What you may also see is that, in some cases, this apparent natural human need for companionship is in reality a need for external acceptance and approval, or is perhaps a superficial cure for the loneliness that comes from not truly being in touch with your inner self. The need for relaxation, too, is a genuine one, and yet true natural relaxation, as we have seen, does not usually result from the kinds of situations and activities that we have come to associate with "relaxation," such as social eating, drinking and group activities.

Experience 15

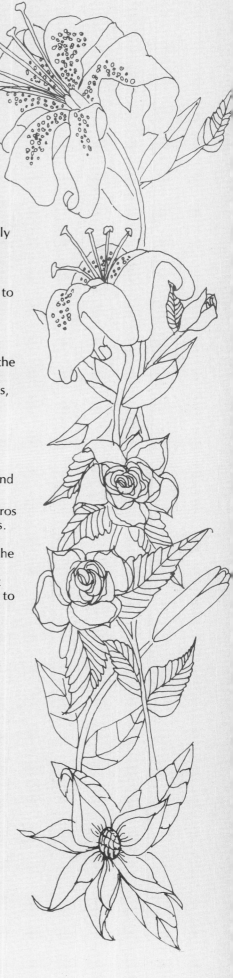

4. Next, ask yourself about each of your social relationships: "Is this relationship a meaningful friendship, which helps both/all of us to grow and learn? Or is it relatively superficial, simply filling the need not to be lonely or to kill time? Does it just exist because we do certain things together? If there weren't any martinis, cups of coffee, gourmet meals, etc., would we still want to spend time with each other? "

These are hard questions to ask of ourselves, and yet, if we want our environment to support our growth in every possible way, we must ask them.

Adjustment

Now it is simply a question of recognizing and accepting your own inner priorities, the urgings of prana as they speak to you through your body and your intuitive feelings. Once you have seen where the conflicts lie in your environment and social situations, you will be able to make the necessary adjustments to your lifestyle.

1. First list the specific changes that you can make easily.

2. Then write down the ways in which you can gradually make other, more difficult changes, while keeping in harmony with those around you.

3. Review the situations in which you cannot realistically make changes at present and resolve to accept them willingly and open-heartedly.

In order to facilitate the above process, it is important to be very clear about the pros and cons of each situation and to weigh them carefully. It's helpful to make two lists. It may be possible to change some things, and yet, all things considered, more desirable *not* to make those changes right now. See where happy compromises are the best solution and where impatience would cause unnecessary difficulties. For example, you might wish as a mother to have all your family become vegetarian, but this could create tremendous strain on the family relationships, so it would be better to simply continue to serve meat. A happy compromise might be to introduce some occasional meat substitutes, excitingly prepared, or to serve more fowl and seafood, de-emphasizing red meat. Everything depends on the situation and the people. The important thing is to be aware of and weigh the possible results of each action.

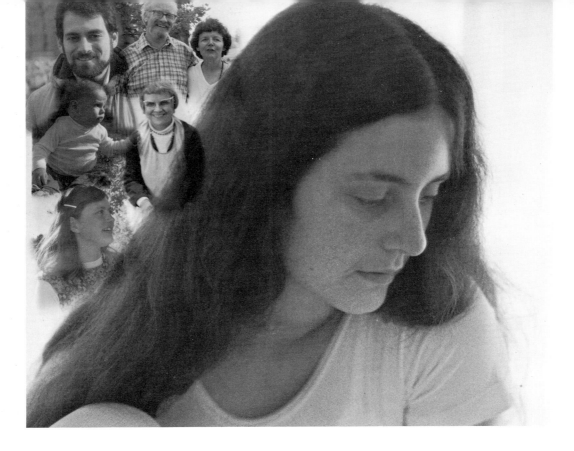

YOUR RELATIONSHIPS

In this article, Yogi Desai talks about how our relationships with those close to us can become more loving and more supportive of our mutual growth.

GIVING AND RECEIVING

by Yogi Amrit Desai

In today's world of self-centered and deteriorating relationships, love has become a very confused and misunderstood concept. Usually what is known as love is no more than attachment. Attachment and love are diametrically opposed qualities. They cannot exist simultaneously; they are mutually exclusive. Love makes no demands; it is free of expectations. We love simply for the sake of loving, for the pure joy of loving in and of itself. Love emanates from the center of peace and contentment which is within us. In attachment, on the other hand, your experience of love depends upon an outside person or object.

In attachment there is a desired result to be gained by loving; there is a goal in the relationship. Attachment is a contract, an exchange. "If you do this, I will love you. If you stop doing it, I will no longer love you." This attachment soon becomes an emotional addiction, a total dependence upon receiving the desired goal. When this goal is not achieved, "love" disappears and pain results.

As two people meet and are attracted to each other, they each discover desirable qualities in the other or needs which they feel can be fulfilled in a mutual relationship. All of the differences which exist between them seem unimportant because the power of emotion is so strong in their relationship. The play of emotional attraction may continue for a long time, particularly during the pre-marriage and early marriage stages. Yet once these powerful emotions begin to settle, the differences begin to be apparent.

If sexual attraction is the glue which holds the relationship together, as the thrill of emotion wanes so also does the relationship. This is because in the temporary strength of sexual union, other areas of growth are often ignored. Sex is unwittingly used as a "cover-up" to temporarily hide arguments or disagreements which develop between the couple-- "Let's kiss and make up." Pain caused by disharmony within the relationship is "swallowed"; resentful anger, disappointment and frustration lodge themselves deep within. Of course, this disharmony can occur within any close relationship. However, marriage is the closest of all relationships, and so communication is considerably more intense.

Loving From Our Inner Center of Contentment

When we truly love we feel compassion for others, but we do not look to them as the means of fulfillment for our emotional needs and addictions. We are aware that happiness is something we draw from the core of our being, and then share with others, not demand from others. This core becomes the source of fulfillment for us. We do not "need" others, in the sense of being totally dependent on them for our happiness. As a result, when we discover and learn to relate from this center of happiness and inner contentment, all who come near us receive our freely given gift of love.

There is only one way to receive love -- and that is to give love. Only when we give freely are we truly able to receive, for in giving we receive inner joy, and this joy is what we really wanted anyway! Many people measure the love they give carefully and watch closely to see if love is returned with equal measure. In truth there is no way we can measure love, for love given with a desire for return is not love -- it is a contract. If we want to be loved, then we must give love totally, with no thought of receiving anything in return. Then we will experience the *state* of love, of being "in love", rather than the act of giving or receiving love.

Love requires continuous practice, and the best place to begin practicing is with ourselves, because everything depends on our own attitude to life. We need to change our habitual attitudes and ways of viewing the world in order to come to that center of inner fulfillment and joy. As we progress in our mastery of love, we can no longer reject anyone simply on the basis of our own value systems or concepts of how they should be. We can no longer entertain negative thoughts about others. Instead, we must begin to live creatively, consciously developing new positive attitudes, habits and experiences.

When difficulties arise between two people, the solution is to begin to actively recall and dwell on the beautiful qualities which we recognize within the other person. As we continue to recall all that we have previously admired and loved in the other person, we discover that our gestures, the words we speak and the way we look at him or her begin to change. He or she instinctively feels our acceptance and love without our ever expressing it in words. Confidence grows within the other that our outlook has become steady and positive, and that they are accepted and loved unconditionally, as they are. Then, the other person also begins to change, and the conflict can be easily resolved.

Words can never disguise a lack of love; that is why we need to change our thinking. If we constantly speak words of love to others and yet entertain negative thoughts; they will not be deceived. They need not be psychologists to read our hidden language. For this reason, it is essential to think only positive thoughts about anyone with whom we are having difficulty. Such positive thinking is not a suppression of negativity; rather, it is a rechanneling process. Negative thoughts are recognized, acknowledged and accepted as natural. Then we simply give them no more attention or energy. As we develop a conscious pattern of honestly recognizing all that we admire within the other person, these positive thoughts will drown out the negative ones just as light dispels the darkness in a room when you turn on the switch. Positive thinking is the major secret of good relations with others.

Marriage For Mutual Growth

A marriage which has as its main purpose the physical, emotional and spiritual growth of the partners enables a deep and lasting union to develop regardless of the outer changing circumstances. As each partner learns to offer support in the most difficult times, as well as in the many times of joy and shared happiness, and works at entertaining only positive feelings about the other partner, the growth which occurs far surpasses any outward support which could be received. Honest and loving faith in each other establishes a chain reaction, for each opportunity in which one part-

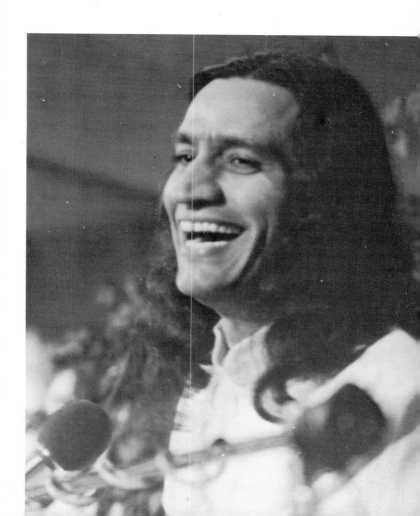

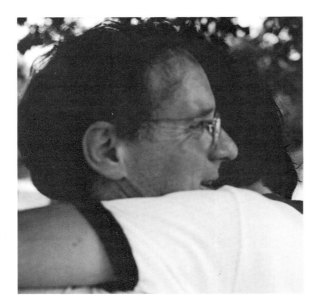

ner can sincerely give enables a warm and sincere exchange of gratitude.

Feelings become totally supportive as each partner strives to be loving in all situations and avoids relying on the other to fulfill his or her emotional needs. Paradoxically enough, all these needs will, in reality, be fulfilled, for the internal happiness and strength which comes from freely giving without expectations brings the experience of deep peace and contentment which was the original basic need anyway. The limited time which modern families are able to spend together will seem to become limitless, for the feeling and togetherness between loving partners will be an ongoing internal experience regardless of the physical distance. Communication becomes loving, honest and open, for there need be no fear as the relationship grows in the power of mutual giving.

Giving Love is Giving Ourselves

When we give love, we are providing security to others. We are caring for them, providing comfort and ease to them. As a result we have no reason to experience tension or anxiety with others because we have made them so secure that they have no reason to do anything we might experience as threatening. When we expect and demand something from others, we subconsciously set up others as a threat, because they are able to withhold whatever we seek from them. As a result, we fear not getting what we need from them and become defensive and self-protective. Thus, providing loving security to others enables us to feel secure. Demanding security from others robs us of the security which is already present within us.

Anyone can create the false feeling of acceptance and belonging by commanding it from some outside source, but only the person of true depth and maturity can find acceptance within. As you learn to accept yourself, to know that you are fine *just as you are,* with all your faults, you will naturally accept your marriage partner and all others with whom you come in contact *as they are.* Only then can you experience and give unconditional love -- love which is free from fear, dependence and attachment. This love can begin by accepting both yourself and others at the same time. Eventually your love will begin to come back to you as you grow in the experience of providing love to others without expectation of return.

It is important to realize that although you can never love too much, you can love too much in your own way, a way which may not be understood by the other person. When you want to love others, you must love in a way that can be accepted and understood by them; a way that they need to receive love. Then they won't feel threatened or imagine that you want something from them and will recognize your love for what it really is -- a free gift.

Simply Drop What Love Is Not

We don't need to know what unconditional love is in order to practice it -- we simply need to know what love is not and to drop those thoughts and actions from our lives. Deep in our hearts, we all know what love is not, what is not loving. It is not loving to hate others, to be jealous of them, to compete with them, to want them to be different than they are. We know that violence is not loving, and so we usually do not perform acts of physical violence. Yet we do not realize that we are constantly performing more subtle acts of "violence" through thoughts and actions which are non-accepting of people (jealousy, competitiveness, the desire to change them). Instead, we can come up with creative solutions to difficult encounters by seeing objectively where we can change our experience of the external situation by changing something in ourselves. This adaptability and willingness to adjust constantly is true unselfishness, which is the very essence of being "loving."

We commit these acts and thoughts of subtle "violence" on ourselves too, every time we reject ourselves, feel guilty or blame ourselves. Only when we are able to first love and accept ourselves *as we are,* unconditionally, will we be able to truly love and accept others.

IN CONCLUSION

As you reach the end of this book, you will have a whole new set of tools to help you progress on the path to Holistic Health. You may feel as if you have made a new friend -- yourself. You will have learned much about this new friend: his/her strengths and beauties, and endearing weaknesses and idiosyncrasies. You will have come to treasure and respect this new friend, in body, mind and spirit. You will be ever amazed and delighted as you daily discover new things about him or her. You will have made this friend some promises, as you would in any relationship. You have promised to always listen to his/her needs, and to try your best to fulfill them. You have committed yourself to doing your utmost to help that friend maintain his/her health, and to lift it to ever higher levels of vibrant well-being. You have promised to relax together, to play together, to share your sorrows and your joys. You have, above all, resolved never to forget or reject this friend, no matter what. For this friend is your very Self.

The appendix, which follows, contains information and suggestions to help you continue your quest for Holistic Health. If you find you have further needs and questions, we warmly invite you to write or call us at the Kripalu Center for Holistic Health. If you would like to deepen and enrich your experience of the techniques we have shared in this book, then consider participating in one of our programs. We have an illustrated catalogue we would be delighted to send you at no charge. You may also like to be on the mailing list for our 16-page, free illustrated newspaper, YOGA QUEST.

We also invite you to send us any feedback you may have on this book. Our whole purpose is to serve you to the very best of our ability, and to do that we need your input.

We will end with the yogic greeting that we use at the Health Center.

JAI BHAGWAN!
(We salute the light within you)

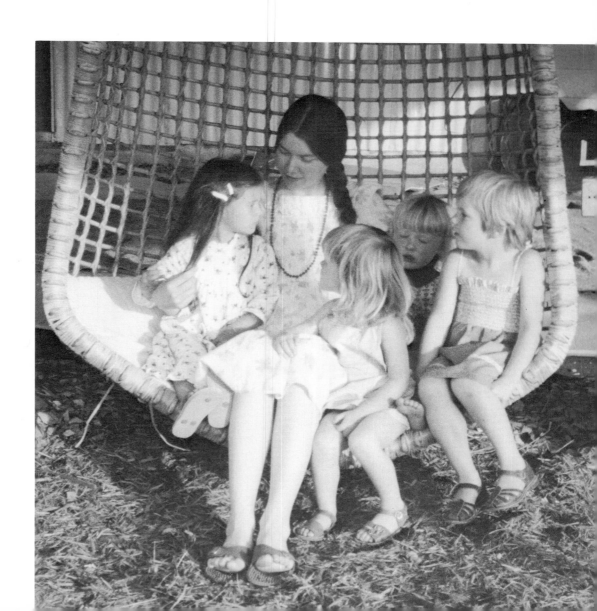

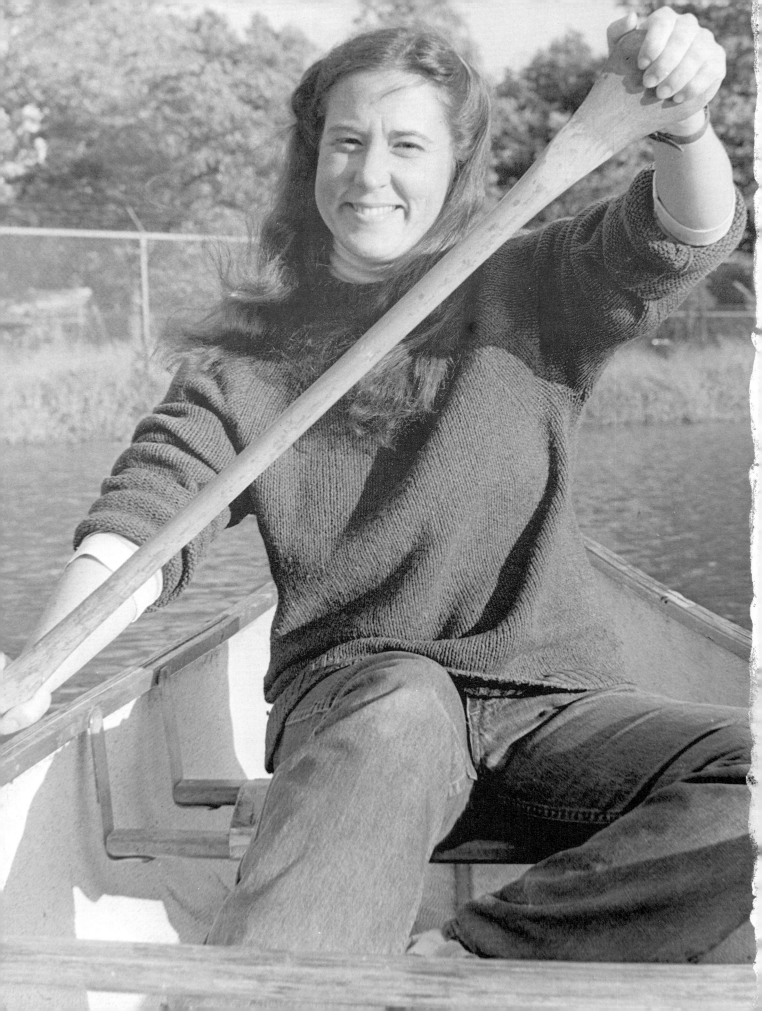

APPENDIX

KRIPALU CENTER FOR YOGA AND HEALTH

Located among the Berkshire mountains of western Massachusetts, Kripalu Center offers year-round educational programs and individual health services which promote holistic health by teaching how to harmonize body, mind and spirit.

The basis of our approach is the time-tested wisdom of yoga and its principle that physical health is the foundation for emotional and spiritual development. Our programs and services combine ancient yoga practices with modern, natural self-development techniques. They provide not just intellectual understanding but also experiential learning and first-hand knowledge of vibrant health and radiant well-being.

Weekend, week-long and four-week programs focus on self-development through yoga, inner awareness, spiritual attunement, fitness and bodywork training. Guests can also individualize their stay, designing their day from a wide selection of classes and other activities.

Individual health services are available both to Center guests and to the general public. These services include sessions in a variety of bodywork techniques such as Shiatsu, polarity, foot and facial care, and Touch for Health™ as well as personal counseling. Our facilities include sauna, whirlpool and floatation tank; a full range of comfortable accommodations; convenient lounges with stunning lake and mountain views; the Kripalu Shop; natural foods kitchen and bakery; spacious rooms for program workshops and daily classes.

Kripalu Center's history traces back to 1966, the year in which Yogi Amrit Desai founded the Yoga Society of Pennsylvania in Philadelphia. By 1969, the Society was sponsoring yoga classes for nearly 2500 students every ten weeks; Yogi Desai personally trained hundreds of yoga teachers to meet the growing demand for yoga classes in the Philadelphia area.

In 1971, Yogi Desai and his family moved from Philadelphia to nearby Sumneytown. Yogi Desai's students sought to continue studying yoga with him and in 1972 a residential community, the Kripalu Ashram, formed at the Sumneytown location.

By 1975, Kripalu Ashram could no longer accommodate the many people who wanted to join the community as residents or the hundreds of guests who wanted to visit. Accordingly, in that year a second property was purchased, which became the Kripalu Yoga Retreat, in Summit Station, Pennsylvania.

The Kripalu Center for Holistic Health was established on the Summit Station property in 1978 to complement the current offerings in yoga and spiritual development with other programs and services promoting holistic health. In just the few years following its origin, the Health Center gained national recognition as one of the best residential holistic health centers in the country.

With thousands of guests visiting the Retreat and Health Center annually, and with many programs fully booked months in advance, Kripalu again sought a larger facility. In December 1983, Kripalu Center for Yoga and Health opened at the present location, in Lenox, Massachusetts.

You can support and extend the benefits this **Self-Health Guide** offers you by visiting Kripalu Center in person and by making use of other books, tapes and products available through the Kripalu Shop. For free program and Kripalu Shop catalogs, write or call: Kripalu Center for Yoga and Health, Box 793, Lenox, MA 01240; (413) 637-3280.

Kripalu Center is a non-profit, federally tax-exempt organization.

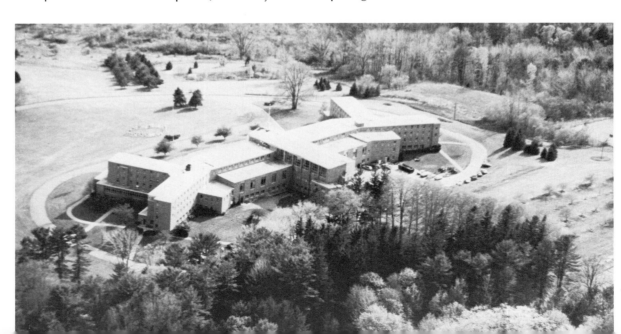

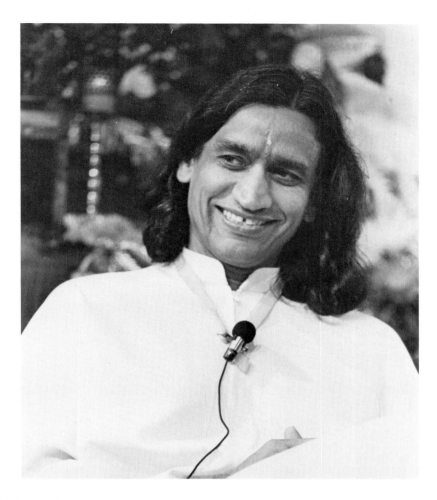

YOGI AMRIT DESAI

Yogi Amrit Desai, founder and spiritual director of Kripalu Center, has devoted more than 35 years to practicing Holistic Health through the science of yoga. His teachings on yoga—one of the most ancient techniques for achieving optimal health and integrating body, mind and spirit—inspire the programs and health services that Kripalu Center offers.

Yogi Desai has received several significant honors, including the rarely-awarded title Doctor of Yoga, and his many achievements have gained international recognition. His most outstanding contribution is his formulation of Kripalu Yoga, a new method of practicing traditional yoga postures for the experience of "meditation in motion". Yogi Desai has also broadened the scope of Kripalu Yoga by expressing it as an all-encompassing approach to living a holistic lifestyle.

As he has developed Kripalu Yoga, Yogi Desai has drawn upon the ancient teachings which he has received from his own spiritual teacher, Swami Shri Kripalvanandji. Swami Kripalvanandji, for whom Kripalu Yoga and the Center are named, is known as one of India's greatest spiritual masters and one of the world's leading exponents of yoga. Yogi Desai's unique achievement is his adaptation of these ancient, esoteric teachings to meet the needs of modern-day Westerners, without in any way sacrificing their purity or authenticity.

Yogi Desai is a well-known and widely travelled lecturer. He has given numerous seminars throughout North America, Europe and India and has appeared several times on national television.

It is Yogi Desai's own presence, however, which speaks most eloquently of the benefits of Kripalu Yoga's holistic approach to living. He is the very model of the healthy, joyful, self-actualizing human being who is living at the peak of his potential. Those who meet him are invariably inspired and energized by his vibrancy, his contagious zest for life, his graceful bearing, his delightful sense of humor. Most of all, people are profoundly touched by his deeply compassionate nature, which reaches out to embrace all he meets with unconditional, warm-hearted acceptance. This compassion and love carry the essence of Yogi Desai's teaching: that the ultimate purpose of Holistic Health is to achieve our highest human potential—to live fully in the experience of love.

INDEX

'4/84-18-BPR-4